Health & Fitness in Plain English

HEALTH & FITNESS

Jolie Bookspan, Ph.D.

in PLAIN ENGLISH

KENSINGTON BOOKS

http://www.kensingtonbooks.com

Nothing in this book is meant as specific medical advice or instruction. See your physician and get training before attempting anything presented.

KENSINGTON BOOKS

are published by

Kensington Publishing Corp.
850 Third Ave.
New York, NY 10022

Copyright © Jolie Bookspan, Ph.D.
Illustrations by Todd Sargood

ISBN 1-57566-288-4

First Printing: June, 1998
10 9 8 7 6 5 4 3 2 1

Printed in the United States of America

THE SURGEON GENERAL
HAS DETERMINED
THAT LACK OF PHYSICAL ACTIVITY
IS DETRIMENTAL
TO YOUR HEALTH.

—*Surgeon General's Report on*
Physical Activity and Health,

July 1996

REVIEWERS

Sincere thanks to the reviewers:

Alan Berg, Ph.D., M.D., *Housecall Doctor. Philadelphia, Pennsylvania.*

Karrie Bookspan, *Aerobics Instructor and Personal Trainer. Florida.*

Russ Gazzara, Ph.D., *Development Neurotoxicologist, National Center for Toxicological Research, FDA. Little Rock, Arkansas.*

Green Beret Lt. Col. R. Kelly Hill, M.D., *Our Lady of the Lake Regional Medical Center, Baton Rouge, Louisiana.*

David Hsu, Ph.D., M.D., *University of Iowa Hospitals and Clinics.*

David Josephson, *Josephson Engineering. San Jose, California.*

David Koeppel, *Writer, Film Editor. Paramount Pictures, Hollywood, California.*

Larry "Scoots" Miller, Ph.D., *Microbiologist. Seattle, Washington.*

Alan Moore, M.D., *Board-Certified, Obstetrics, Gynecology, and Family Medicine, The Woodlands, Texas (Chapter 22).*

Rich Ruoti, Ph.D., P.T., P.C., *BuxMont Physical Therapy, Warminster, Pennsylvania (Chapters 20 and 21).*

Audrey Tannenbaum, M.Ed., A.T.C., C.S.C.S., *Athletic Trainer and Maccabean Games Triathlon Gold Medalist. Horsham, Pennsylvania.*

Marla Tonseth, P.T., M.B.A., *Physical Therapist, Private Practice. Warrington, Pennsylvania (Chapters 20 and 21).*

William B. Young, M.D., *Jefferson Headache Center, Thomas Jefferson University Hospital, Philadelphia, Pennsylvania (Chapter 29).*

CONTENTS

Part II—Nutrition

Part III—Health

What's in This Book

Finally. A book on health, nutrition, and fitness, all together, and written in plain English. This book is for everyone, regardless of physical condition or academic background.

Topics in each chapter were selected from questions people ask most frequently. In nontechnical language this book puts solid information in the place of myths; details hundreds of fun, upbeat ideas for exercise, health, and nutrition; explains the mysterious terminology of fitness; and gives step-by-step suggestions for healthier living. It's all here, from how to lose weight; to what to do about back pain, headaches, osteoporosis, and leg cramps; to what do good and bad cholesterol mean, and how you can control your own levels. There are answers to those fun little questions about our bodies that everyone wonders about, like why does your foot fall asleep? Why do your joints crackle and pop? Why does it hurt so much to ding your funny bone? At the end of the book, there is a large, annotated glossary. More than a handy reference of definitions, it includes word derivations, key concepts, and fun stories behind the people and information.

With the information in this book you will be better equipped to make sense of the many claims and counterclaims in exercise, health, and nutrition. You will be better prepared to start your exercise program—and stay on it. You will be able to make informed decisions about your health. You'll even have fun.

Happy reading.

Part One

Exercise

A vigorous five-mile walk will do more good for an unhappy but otherwise healthy adult than all the medicine and psychology in the world.

—Paul Dudley White

1

Why Should You Get Fit?

*I don't exercise. What's in it for me? You've got to offer
me more than my life to get me on a Stairmaster grunting
for two hours. I view my body as a way of getting my
head from one place to another.*

—Dave Thomas, founder of Wendy's

Good physical condition is important for everyone. This is true even
if you are not an athlete. Good fitness reduces your risk of many
serious diseases, delays several common effects of aging, increases
your tolerance to heat and cold, increases muscle, and reduces fat.
Regular exercise, and the wellness it brings, helps you cope with
stress and feel better in general. Good physical fitness can improve
your safety and comfort during your daily life and recreational activities. How is this all so?

Better Health

An active lifestyle makes major positive changes in your health and
well-being. Common Western ills, such as heart and blood vessel
disease, obesity, some types of diabetes, and many musculoskeletal
problems, are known as *hypokinetic* diseases (*hypo*- means "less than"
or "not enough," and *kinetic* means "activity"). *Hypokinetic disease*

is a fancy term for illness related to, or even caused by, being sedentary and out of shape.

- Epidemiologic studies suggest that regular exercise lowers incidence of breast cancer in women, and colon and reproductive tract cancer risk in both men and women.
- Resistance exercise thickens bones, important osteoporosis prevention (Chapter 22).
- Cardiovascular fitness through aerobic exercise reduces your risk of early death from vascular disease, heart disease, and high blood pressure, all major killers of both men and women (Chapter 27).
- Sudden death from heart attack is more common in an out-of-shape person who exerts past capacity, than in those who regularly exercise.

Delayed Aging

Although your chronological years increase, you can become functionally younger with exercise. It's difficult to separate the toll of aging from just sitting around too much. Still, getting slower and weaker as years pass is not solely an inescapable aging process. To varying degrees, it comes from not enough activity.

Your body functions decline predictably both with aging and without enough physical activity:

- As years pass without exercise, your muscular strength, speed, and power all drop off sharply.
- After about age thirty, the deterioration would run about 0.75% to 1% per year if you didn't regularly exercise.
- The maximum amount of oxygen your body can use to make energy, an important indicator of fitness, would drop about 10% each decade from ages 20 to 60.
- Without flexibility exercises, joints tighten with passing years until ordinary reaching and bending can become difficult, and in many cases, impossible.

Regular exercise and stretching considerably slows, even reverses, all this loss in many cases, meaning gains equivalent to stopping or reversing years of aging. Older people who exercise and stretch have many of the functional characteristics of a chronologically younger person. They can reach and run and move easily. The anti-aging effect of exercise is possible for all age groups. Geriatric populations on exercise programs considerably improve strength and mobility. Often physical gains are enough to remove their need for walkers, wheelchairs, and canes. They improve their self-sufficiency so much that once again, they can carry out their own activities of daily living. All from regular exercise.

Fewer, Less Serious Injuries

Better physical fitness may lower your risk of joint injury during regular physical activity. Pushing beyond capacity, which is easy to do when you don't have much capacity to begin with, can easily lead to pain and overuse injuries. Lt. Col. Bruce H. Jones, M.D., Chief of the Occupational Medicine Division of the U.S. Army Research Institute of Environmental Medicine, reported on data from army recruits. He found that those of lower physical fitness had consistently higher injury rates than those of higher fitness.

Good joint flexibility seems to be important to reduce injuries. A tight-jointed exerciser may have a higher incidence of muscle pulls and strains. A person with tight back muscles is back pain waiting to happen. Although men usually have less natural flexibility than women, particularly of the lower extremities where injury rates are high, men can attain healthful flexibility with regular stretching. It is not true that having big muscles or lifting weights reduces flexibility; lack of stretching reduces flexibility. More on flexibility in Chapter 6.

Everyone needs physical exercise for general health and injury prevention. Without it, a vicious cycle of inactivity and injury grows. If you are sedentary, begin to become more active slowly and carefully, working within your safety and comfort zone to make activity a lifetime habit, rather than a chore to endure and avoid if possible.

Positive Mood

Regular exercise is thought to affect your mood positively in several ways.

- In the short term, a vigorously exercising body is thought to manufacture a class of hormones called endorphins, although specifics are far from established. The word *endorphin* is a contraction of "endogenous [made from within] morphine-like substance." It's not definitely known, but feasible, that endorphins improve mood after hard workouts by releasing chemicals that stimulate your brain's pleasure center.

- In the long term, and more firmly accepted, exercise increases your overall fitness so that you can do things you enjoy more often and more comfortably.
- Regular exercise is established to reduce premenstrual symptoms and cramping during menses.
- Regular exercise helps decrease the moodiness and sugar cravings that often strike in the late afternoons, by increasing insulin sensitivity. That means less insulin mobilizes to process a given load of carbohydrate. This seems to be the case no matter what time of day you exercise, as long as you exercise regularly. Your blood sugar maintains a steadier level, reducing the swings that produce food cravings and moodiness.
- Regular exercise seems to be associated with reduced symptoms of depression and anxiety.
- Greater physical ability, body awareness, and improved body shape and health with exercise might also make you happy. Overall, the specifics of how exercise improves your emotional state are not clearly mapped. Still, there is evidence for a relationship between long-term exercising and an increased feeling of well-being and ability to face emotional stress.

Reduced Fatigue

It may seem backward that exercising can make you less tired, and not exercising can leave you tired. But exercise works to reduce your overall levels of fatigue.

- The out-of-shape body doesn't use oxygen efficiently. When your body can't supply the oxygen that your muscles demand, you tire easily doing ordinary activities.
- Out-of-shape muscles find it tiring to do simple tasks that strong muscles can easily accomplish.
- Regular exercise raises your body's level of physical "readiness," making you feel more energetic.
- A brisk walk or other short exercise can "pick you up" more than a candy bar.

- Regular exercise makes many physical changes in your body, including more blood volume and oxygen-carrying blood cells, better strength and tone of your various body parts, and other changes that make you feel energetic.

A vicious cycle occurs when you are too out-of-shape to exercise enough to get much exercise benefit. Sitting around makes you tired and weak, which reduces your ability and inclination to exercise.

A positive cycle comes about when you stick with an exercise program until you become accustomed to regular exercise, and can exercise hard enough to make gains, which in turn, allows you to do more and feel better and more energetic.

Better Tolerance to Heat

Exercise in the heat has been described as probably the single greatest stress ever imposed on the human cardiovascular system. When you improve your physical fitness, your body makes changes that improve your ability to tolerate heat and do activity in the heat.

Blood supply to your heart and limb muscles is crucial for you to move around. You also need to shunt blood to your skin to take heat away from your body to cool you. Because there is only a finite amount of blood to go around, competition can develop.

- A fitter person has more total body fluid volume, including blood volume, and can pump more blood with each heartbeat.
- The fitter person can supply blood to muscles for movement and skin for cooling, without running short for either one.
- Fitter people increase how much they can sweat for cooling.
- With increased fluids to go around for cooling, body core temperature will not rise as high at the same exercise intensity as in an out-of-shape person.
- The out-of-shape person has less cooling capacity, and decreased ability to do activities safely in the heat.

More than any other factor, physical fitness reduces your susceptibility to overheating. If you get out of shape, you lose your adaptations. Improved fitness, and the improved heat tolerance that comes with it, is not only for athletes who exercise in the heat, but for everyone who spends any time in the heat.

Better Tolerance to Cold

Physical fitness improves tolerance to exercise in cold environments, although to a much lesser extent than for heat tolerance. Even so, the structural and metabolic changes that occur with regular exercise appear to keep you warmer in the cold:

- Increased muscle mass, which you would get through resistance exercise, increases heat production and storage.
- A fit person can do more exercise to keep warm in the cold.
- A fit person tolerates a lower body temperature than an unfit person before shivering starts.

Exercise in the cold improves your cold tolerance much more than exercise alone.

Recreational Fun and Safety

A high degree of muscular strength, cardiovascular endurance, and muscular endurance positively affects your capacity for exertion common to many activities you enjoy for sport and for health. You call on your exercise reserves for extended efforts like long runs, roller blading, biking, and swimming; shorter, more intense efforts like a few hard matches of tennis; or the changing demands of a weekend hike, carrying groceries or kids, or doing household chores.

- Someone with high cardiovascular capacity can more easily run, hike, or swim a distance that is hard work to someone with less cardiovascular adaptation.
- Better fitness makes daily chores around the house and yard easier.
- Fitter people perceive less exertion at the same exercise intensity so they can do more before pooping out.
- Fitter people are less likely to have heart trouble during activities.

Being in good condition may make the difference between a difficult situation and an easy jaunt.

Fat Loss

Exercise burns calories so you can lose weight, or even eat more without gaining weight. Regular exercise burns fat and shifts your body to a mode where it burns more fat for fuel in general and during exercise. When your body preferentially burns fat, it extends the supply of the carbohydrates stored in your muscles and liver, thereby extending your exercise capacity.

Getting "in Shape" vs. Getting Healthy

You hear all the confusing recommendations—some sources say you need five days a week of hard exercise, others claim you need only three days a week of moderate exercise. The answer is simple. Different levels of exercise will give you different levels of results. Mild to moderate exercise three days a week will begin to improve your health. Your disease risks will begin to go down, and you will start feeling and looking better. Exercising more vigorously and more often makes bigger changes. This does not mean you have to kill yourself. Overdoing exercise will not get you much more gain than regular, vigorous exercise, but increases your risk of injury.

The *Surgeon General's Report on Physical Activity and Health* released in 1996 defines moderate exercise as using about 150 calories per day, or 1,000 calories a week. This is about a half hour of medium-intensity exercise per day.

You don't even need to go to a gym. Be active as a way of daily life, in a variety of ways, and you need never see the inside of a gym.

It Pays

Being in good physical condition is important to your life, even if you never intend to play sports or climb mountains. The many health and well-being payoffs contribute to safe, healthful, and fun living every day.

2

The Different Aspects of Fitness

You've got to be very careful if you don't know where you are going, because you might not get there.

—Yogi Berra

There are different ways you can be in shape. You need to know the different aspects of fitness so that you can know where you're going with your fitness program. Each different fitness aspect needs different types of exercise. Without exercising each in its own way, you "might not get there."

Why Different Aspects of Fitness?

Swimming, walking, and jogging increase your cardiovascular (aerobic) endurance, but not your strength. Dashing around playing tennis, or other sprint activity, doesn't improve your ability to go long distances. Taking long daily walks or runs will not build big muscles. Neither will sit-ups take fat off your stomach; for that you need aerobic work. Weight lifting is usually not aerobic exercise, despite what health clubs tell you. Stretching makes you more flexible, not stronger. Why?

Cardiovascular endurance, anaerobic capacity, muscular strength, power, and muscular endurance are different body systems, both structurally and chemically. Different activities make different adaptations in your different systems, giving you different kinds of fitness. To walk or run long distances, you need to train for distance. It also means that being fit in only one way won't be as much help to the other things you need to do. For lifting grocery bags, strong biceps (among other muscles), separate those people struggling from those lifting easily. Big biceps won't help your swimming, because swimming doesn't use the biceps much. To get the effect you want, you need to do the right training. This chapter tells the interesting story behind each specific adaptation to different exercise. Then Chapter 3 tells specifically how to improve each aspect of your fitness.

Flexibility

Power

Strength

Cardiovascular and
muscular endurance

Anaerobic capacity

Figure 2.1. There are several components to fitness. You need them all, not just for sports, but for your everyday life.

Cardiovascular Endurance (Aerobic Capacity)

Cardiovascular endurance is also called cardiorespiratory endurance or aerobic capacity. It's the ability of your heart and lungs and their interconnected system of blood vessels to supply oxygen and nutrients to the parts that move you around. Your body uses this oxygen to make energy, so the process is called *aerobic,* which means "with oxygen."

Your cardiovascular endurance determines how long you can walk, run, bike, dance, skate, ski, jog, or swim at your chosen pace. It contributes to how tired you will be at the end of doing things you need to do all day. It affects your general health. Improving your aerobic condition makes getting where you want to go easier, and means you can get through your day more easily and with less fatigue. *See* Chapter 4, "What Does 'Aerobic' Really Mean?" for the details on what it means to be aerobic.

Anaerobic Capacity

Not all activities are aerobic. With fast activity, your body doesn't have a chance to activate its aerobic system. Your body has to use quick and ready-stored fuel, not oxygen, so this activity is called *an*aerobic. *Anaerobic* means "without oxygen." You barely have enough stored energy for a few minutes of anaerobic activity. If you continue activity at a pace that is too fast for you, your body can't switch over to its oxygen-using aerobic system to any great extent. Your body continues trying to use your stored fuel. But your demand exceeds the supply, and you run out of fuel. If you won't slow down so that your body can switch to the aerobic system that can make more energy, your body will stop you, gasping, in your tracks—anaerobic.

You use your anaerobic system to run for a bus, get out of your chair, lift packages, throw things, do things holding your breath like swimming underwater, and do any short, hard activity. Developing your anaerobic system will make all these activities easier and safer. If your body is not prepared for short, quick activities, you can wind up hurting yourself. Your anaerobic system is explained more in Chapter 4, "What Does 'Aerobic' Really Mean?"

Strength

Muscular strength is usually measured by the maximum force your muscles can generate in a single effort. You need strength to lift and carry weights, packages, and yourself easily, rather than struggle. By increasing your strength through weight lifting, you can move around more easily, and reduce your chance of musculoskeletal injury while doing it.

Some elderly and debilitated people who could not previously even lift themselves out of their chairs became more mobile after strengthening programs, allowing them to walk unaided once again.

Some people believe that women should not do weight lifting (for any number of reasons, including the fear of getting large muscles). Weight lifting is important for women's health. Even women who don't do activities commonly regarded as strength activities, need strength to do daily activities like carrying several 20 pound grocery bags and a 40+ pound child. Weight lifting to increase muscular strength also strengthens bones. The pull of muscle against bone thickens the bone. The stronger a muscle, the more it can pull on the bones it attaches to. Weight lifting is a key part of osteoporosis prevention.

Weight lifting to strengthen muscles also thickens bones, helping prevent osteoporosis.

Extra muscle helps you stay warm in winter, and is your chief calorie burner. Building more muscle through strength training means that you burn more calories every day.

Every pound of muscle you gain through strength training increases your metabolic rate by about 50 calories per day.
If you gain five pounds of muscle, you burn about 250 more calories every day, even when just sitting around.

Power

In exercise physiology, power is measured by how fast you can be strong. It's a product of speed and strength together. You call on power to lift things, throw things, move things, dash out of the way of cars, or catch a falling child or package.

Different activities need different amounts of strength compared to speed. To throw the discus and lob a tennis ball, you take a light weight and hurl it fast and far away. Offensive linemen try to do the same to heavy defensive backs and tackles. A higher strength component compared to how fast you move, for example in bench pressing or lifting any weight, is called strength-dominated power. Swimming, running, jumping, and tennis, use primarily speed-dominated power.

Power is not just for athletes. When you increase your power, you can move things and yourself around more quickly and easily, with less chance of injury while doing it.

Muscular Endurance

Walking, jogging, biking, skating, and swimming involve many, many leg or arm repetitions against the relatively light resistance of the ground, the bicycle pedal, or the water. High repetitions against low resistance call on muscular endurance.

Muscular endurance is different from cardiovascular endurance. It is just endurance of the specific muscles you are working, not your heart and aerobic system. Untrained muscles do not have muscular endurance. They will get tired before you are out of breath. Trained muscles have specific changes in their cells and how they function that increase endurance capacity. These adaptations don't change muscle size.

Improved muscular endurance makes long walks, runs, rides, and swims easier, and reduces your chance of leg cramps. For carrying things around, and just getting through the day, muscular endurance of your back muscles can make the difference between an uneventful day, and a tired, achy back that night.

Flexibility

Flexibility is the ability to move easily and safely through a range of motion. You need good flexibility to reach shelves and cabinets, bend to tie your shoes and pick things up, and safely do recreational activities.

Several body areas appear susceptible to injury from poor flexibility. The range of motion required to strain tight low-back muscles is quite small, accounting for many painful backs. With good flexibility, you may suffer fewer injuries to your muscles and the tough fibrous structures called tendons that attach your muscles to your bones.

Regular stretching reduces many problems of poor posture and tight, achy joints. *See* Chapter 6, "Stretching and the Six Great Stretching Mistakes."

Aspects of Fitness

Cardiovascular Endurance, also called aerobic fitness. Ability of your heart and lungs, and their system of blood vessels, to supply oxygen and nutrients to the parts that move you around. Enables you to run, swim, bike, skate, walk, ski, and dance farther and longer, with less effort.

Anaerobic Capacity. Stored fuel system for short, intense activity. Enables you to run or swim short distances quickly, exert against resistances like pushing open a stuck door, and do strenuous exercise.

Strength. Ability to move a heavy weight once, or a few times. Increasing your strength makes it easier to lift weights and yourself around.

Muscular Endurance. Ability to move a light weight repeatedly. You need muscular endurance of the legs to walk, jog, and cycle long distances and to go dancing all night. You need muscular endurance of your arms to swim.

Power. Ability to move weight quickly. You call on power to push, pull, punch, throw, and lift things and yourself quickly.

Flexibility. Ability to move easily and safely through a range of motion. Healthy flexibility—not too much, not too little—can reduce pulls and strains.

Not Just One

You need all the different aspects of fitness for a healthy, comfortable life. Doing only one sport or exercise that develops only one aspect of fitness is robbing you, and possibly setting the stage for health problems. The next chapter explains how to develop each different aspect of fitness.

3

Improving Your Fitness

Speaking generally, all parts of the whole body which have a function, if used in moderation and exercised in labors to which each is accustomed, become thereby healthy and well developed, and age slowly; but if unused and left idle, they become liable to disease, defective in growth, and age quickly.

—Hippocrates

A little over 2,500 years ago, the Greek athlete Milo realized he could increase strength by using workloads above those normally encountered. He began lifting a young calf every day. The calf's maturing weight provided progressive resistance until, it was said, he carried the grown bull around the Olympic arena. He became a military hero, and as an Olympic wrestler was undefeated.

Whether Milo lifted an increasingly heavy calf is legend or fact, it is well established that fitness improves by progressively increasing the load, a process called overload. Routinely carrying increasingly heavy loads, for example, increases strength. Progressively raising the number of times you lift a light weight improves muscular endurance. Progressively swimming farther extends your cardiovascular endurance. Increasing your joint range of motion improves your flexibility.

Thin people can be out of shape. Average-weight people can be out of shape. Fat people can be in or out of shape but still want to drop some fat. Even athletic people can be out of shape. Understanding differences among aspects of fitness was covered in the previous chapter. This chapter covers how to improve each of your different aspects of fitness, so you can get in the shape you want.

Cardiovascular Endurance

You can improve your cardiovascular status through continuous low-intensity large muscle activity like walking, running, skating, dancing, biking, cross-country skiing, and swimming.

If your activity is too hard for your fitness level, you will get out of breath and need to stop, cutting the aerobic benefits short. If your intensity is too low, as in slow walking, or exercise class "floor work" of leg lifts and abdominal crunches, you also will not gain aerobic exercise benefit (or burn as many calories). Keep an easy moderate pace.

Exercise studies find a close match between how hard your body actually works and how hard you consider the activity. That means you can easily monitor your workload. A pace you find to be medium effort usually is a medium load on your system, and is about right for exercising for general cardiovascular fitness. A good rule of thumb is to be able to carry on a conversation. If you are too out of breath to talk, you are working at an intensity that is too high to be mostly aerobic. See the next chapter, "What Does 'Aerobic' Really Mean?" for more on this interesting subject.

Recommendations call for regular moderate exercise to improve your health. But what is moderate?
Luckily your body is smart. Exercise that feels moderate is moderate. Exercise that feels too easy really is too easy.

Anaerobic Capacity

You need good anaerobic capacity to get you through short hard exertions, anything from dashing to catch a bus, to rushing up a flight of stairs, to throwing a ball. Improve your anaerobic capacity through high-intensity, short-duration activity like sprint runs and swims, and going up stairs. Alternate sprints with rests.

Gradually work up to 30 seconds of hard anaerobic work, then 1 minute of aerobic "rest," which is easy, mild activity, until your heart rate returns to normal. Then increase the times and the repetitions, keeping the 1:2 ratio of anaerobic work to active rest.

As with aerobic activity, you can tell your intensity by how it feels.

You are anaerobic when you are working hard and fast enough to be out of breath, and the workload feels taxing, even uncomfortable. Train for this, and what was previously uncomfortable becomes possible, and eventually easy.

Strength

Strength training is good for you. Some people reject lifting for fear of hurting themselves or becoming bulky. Done properly, strength training makes you look trimmer and reduces your chance of injury from other activities. It increases your ability to do the physical work of any of your favorite activities, firms your muscles, strengthens your joints, and increases your amount of muscle, which burns calories and keeps you warm. Lifting weights is an important part of osteoporosis prevention, because the stress of muscle pulling against bone increases bone density.

Weight lifting increases bone density, important to prevent thinning bones.

Your body makes several adaptations to increase your strength when you start a weight-lifting program for strength. Usually the first adaptation is a learning effect, which immediately increases the amount you can lift, even before any physical changes occur in your muscles. Then, three physical changes begin. The firing rate of nerves serving your muscles increases, the number of nerve-muscle units, called motor units, that can fire together increase, and you increase the size (cross-sectional area) of your muscle.

For the first three to four weeks, it is the neural factors that predominate to increase your strength. After that, strength increases in young males primarily by increasing size of the muscle. Women and older men increase strength more through neural mechanisms than size, even when they make the same strength increases as a young man. Obviously women and older men can increase muscle size through training, but size is not the only predictor of strength. Strong things may come in small packages.

How Do Your Muscles Get Stronger?

1. The firing rate of nerves serving your muscles increases.
2. More nerve-muscle units can fire together.
3. Your muscle cells themselves get bigger.

Because maximum strength contributes to winning specific Olympic events and—even more crucial—football games, studies have subjected strength training methods to microscopic scrutiny. It has been found that to get stronger you need to contract muscles at close to the maximum they are able to contract. That takes heavy weight, and is why most exercise class "floor work" does not strengthen. Your leg is not heavy enough. You need a weight that is so heavy that after 8–10 lifts you are just about unable to lift it again. It's almost heretical to say swimming won't make you strong. Like floor work without weights in exercise classes, water is not heavy enough to make your muscles work maximally after only 8–10 strokes. That doesn't mean swimming and water exercises are not good for you in other ways. It means they are not major strength builders unless you are debilitated from sickness or injury, or do large numbers of laps at high speeds, which increase your intensity and total work.

Most studies agree the maximum number of times to consecutively lift a heavy weight to maximize strength gain is between 4 and 10 repetitions or "reps." These same studies find less gain with more or fewer reps. Why? If you can do more reps with the same amount of weight, you are not using a weight heavy enough for maximum strength gain. Fewer reps also don't sufficiently overload a muscle to gain strength. Strength work will "tone" or firm you up more than leg lifts or arm circles, which are high repetitions using light weights.

What about recommendations for weight lifting that say to do 8–12 repetitions? That also works. It will not maximize strength building quite so much, but it uses a slightly lighter weight, making the activity safer. For the recreational lifter, the 8–12 repetition recommendation is probably preferable. For the serious strength builder, who has good training and supervision, the heavier weight, fewer repetition recommendation better applies.

One group of repetitions is called a *set*. Slowly and safely work up to three sets of repetitions. But start easy. Try one set to start. After a week or so, if this easy start produces no pain or other problems, increase gradually until you can comfortably do two to three sets. Lift the weight through as complete a range of motion as is comfortable. Control the weight to avoid risk of injury.

How to Train to Get Stronger

1. Carefully experiment to find the heaviest weight that you can comfortably and safely lift 4–8 times (repetitions) for serious, supervised strength building, or 8–12 repetitions for a general strengthening program.
2. Work up to three sets of repetitions.
3. Rest 1–4 minutes between each set.

Between each set, you need rest. Rest allows you to recover enough to maximize muscular tension for the next set. A rest of 1–4 minutes between each set is usually enough. Allow a minimum of a full day between weight training sessions for muscle repair and strength building processes to proceed without interference. When you have progressed to where you can easily lift the weight for three sets, increase the weight.

Balance is important, that is, strengthening muscles that are opposite each other. For example, strengthening your abdominal muscles without also strengthening your back muscles opposite them often causes your "abs" to chronically pull your torso with more tension than your back muscles; the result is back pain and poor posture. Chapters 20 and 21 cover back pain and back exercises.

Many people exercise their abdominal muscles, then never contract their back muscles to strengthen them, too.
Poor posture and back pain often result.
It is ironic that so many gyms and "health" clubs have "abs only" classes.

What about eating more protein to get stronger? Many popular fitness magazines sell protein supplements, stating you need extra protein to build muscle. This is rarely true. The Western diet usually provides much more protein than you need, even with heavy activity. You ordinarily do not need to eat additional protein to increase strength or musculature. Making sure you eat enough carbohydrate to fuel your exercise has been found to help. Not getting enough carbohydrate is fatiguing. For more on healthy eating, *see* Chapter 18.

Lifting is important to everyone's fitness plan. It's a myth that being strong reduces your coordination or flexibility. You can be strong with poor coordination, but not too strong.

It is not true that if you stop exercising, your muscles will turn to fat. Your muscle cells will shrink, as with any other "use-it-or-lose-it" situation, but they cannot transform into a different cell.

Muscular Endurance

Muscular endurance is the ability of any particular muscle or muscle group to continuously do activity at low intensity. Examples are found any time you exert against light weights many times, as with leg lifts, pedaling a bicycle, swimming, or walking. Training is simple. When you have progressed to where you can easily continue for a set number of kicks, strokes, reps, or minutes, increase them gradually. Alternate easy and hard workouts, rest adequately, and don't overdo. The long duration, low intensity, large muscle aspect of training for muscular endurance also increases cardiovascular endurance to varying degrees.

Power

Power is the product of strength and speed. Lifting a weight takes strength. Throwing a weight takes power.

You increase your muscular power any time you move faster against a given load, get stronger, or both in varying combinations. To develop power, lift or move a weight (a package, a dumbbell, or yourself) that you customarily need to lift or move, but do it more quickly. There are special weight machines specifically made for power training.

Be extremely careful when training with weights for power. The potential for serious injury throwing weights around is high. Never lean over and lift quickly unless you really want to ruin your back.

Developing power for swimming or running is safer. Increase your swimming or running power by swimming or running hard every few laps. Rest with easy laps. Be sure to be well warmed up before beginning power laps. While you're at the pool, you can practice throwing a rescue line to increase your throwing power. Lift yourself out of the pool without using the ladder to improve your lifting power. It can also be a cool-looking way to get out of the pool.

Flexibility

Stretching increases the range of joint motion you need for daily mobility, not just for sports. There is good evidence that good flexibility prevents muscle injuries and reduces back pain.

Although stretching for flexibility can reduce injuries, stretching wrong can produce them, by loosening your joints until they don't seat well, thereby increasing wear and tear. Excessive joint laxity predisposes you to sprains and dislocations. Lax shoulder capsules may allow the bones of your shoulder joint to slip out of place from forces that healthier joint capsules tolerate. Good forward and backward ankle flexibility is important for general pain-free walking, and for many sports, particularly swimming, but excess looseness on the outsides of your ankles increases your chance of ankle sprains because your ankle can bend at a high angle sideways if you stumble. Chapter 6 on stretching details what you need for healthy flexibility.

Proper flexibility reduces your chance of muscle and joint injuries and reduces back pain.
Bad stretching exercises can increase your chance of injury by destabilizing joints.

Better exercise education and instructor certification programs have reduced the use of several problematic exercises and stretches. But many unhealthy practices are still with us. To keep your stretching healthful, avoid the following still-common, incorrect stretching practices:

- Don't stretch cold muscles; warm up first. Warming up literally means increasing your body temperature. At cooler muscle temperatures, it takes less force and stretch to tear muscle fibers. Activities that warm you enough to safely begin exercise are large muscle exercises like pedaling a bicycle or slow jogging. Stretching doesn't raise your body temperature, so it's not a warm-up.
- Hold your position for about 30 seconds without bouncing.
- Forget "No pain, no gain." Stretching shouldn't hurt.
- Several well-known stretches hold the joint at an angle that puts too much weight and pressure on ligaments. The hurdler's stretch is a major example. It twists your knee sideways. Instead, keep the nonstretched leg in front of you with your foot on the floor. Clasping hands behind you, then lifting your arms strains the front, and weakest part, of your shoulder capsule. Squatting on your heels is tough on knee ligaments by prying the knee slightly apart, particularly if you have heavy legs. Full squatting can damage the small cartilaginous cushions in your knees, called meniscus. The bad knees of professional baseball catchers come from chronic squatting. Avoid neck ligament stretchers like the "plow" which involves lying with your legs in the air over your head and much weight on your neck, lengthening it forward. A stretch that puts too much weight on your spine occurs when you bend over from a stand for toe touching or worse—bouncing while bending over for toe touching. The groin stretch, sitting with knees bent and soles of the feet touching, can overstretch the side of the ankles if the sides of the feet are left on the floor, rather than kept in line with the lower leg.
- Avoid stretching in one direction without countering the stretch in the other. A common example is stretching forward through toe touching and abdominal crunches, without also stretching the other way by arching backward. Chronic forward bending, particularly with no countering backward stretching is tough on the discs in your spine. A typical result of unbalanced stretching is often seen in dancers who stretch their legs outward without equal stretching inward. The outside of their legs gradually tightens and shortens while the inside loosens until they walk like ducks. Later their hips and knees succumb to early wear. Another example you've probably seen is round-shouldered muscle men. They build up the chest without stretching it, and neglect the back except to allow it to stretch through

slouching. A problem results called stretch-weakness. Their backs cannot counter the pull of their strong and shortened big chests.

- To stretch safely, warm up enough to sweat before you stretch. Then stretch by slowly easing into, then holding the stretch. Don't bounce. Micro-injuries can result. Keep the limb you're stretching in line with the joint to stretch the muscle, not the ligaments. To stretch your hamstrings without hurting your back, lie on your back, bend both knees with your feet on the floor. Leave one foot on the floor and straighten the other leg overhead. To avoid posture problems and back pain from unequal stretching, practice safe backs during stretching: Stretch your upper back, lower back, and hip in each natural direction. Don't overweight your neck by putting your body weight on it. Do sitting and lying-down stretches instead of standing bent over stretches. During the rest of the day avoid sitting with a rounded back. Keep the normal inward curve of your lower back.

Don't stretch by bending over to touch your toes from a
stand. Stretch sitting or lying down instead. When
sitting, keep the normal inward curve of your lower back,
and lean forward from the hip, not your back or neck.
Do only one leg at a time.

Increasing muscle size to the extent that bodybuilders do is not a specific aspect of fitness. Since the topic of gaining size is of high interest, both to those who want it and to those who worry that exercise will make them big, the topic of size is covered here.

An unfortunate number of women, and even men, shun weight lifting and its associated health benefits on the assumption they will grow huge. But gaining an appreciable amount of size takes a lot of work—more than many people are willing to do. You can lift weights to get strong, build endurance, gain power, and become healthy. You will get firm and look good, but you won't bulk up big without specific and intense work.

One look at power lifters and you know they're strong. Yet they look different from bodybuilders. Power lifters train for strength; bodybuilders maximize size and visual effect. Two things bodybuilders do differently are to increase volume of work and muscle definition.

Power lifters and bodybuilders look different even though they both train by lifting heavy weights. They train differently, and get different results for that reason.

Volume is the product of how much weight you lift and how many times you lift it. To maximize volume, do more reps and more sets. Lift more slowly than you would for strength or power. You still need heavy weight, but to be able to do more reps, use less weight than for strength training. Use a weight you can lift 12 or so times before muscle failure stops you. Do more sets and take only short rests between those sets. When you can easily lift 4 sets of 12, increase the weight and, later on, add another set. Definition comes from losing fat under the skin that covers your nooks and crannies.

Someone with large muscles may not be able to lift as much weight in a single effort as a smaller person who trained specifically for strength. It's difficult to make true assessments about the strength of women or older men, or anyone for that matter, purely on muscle circumference.

Firm

Like size, body firmness is not a component of fitness or necessary for health. But since most weight lifting will firm you, and so many people's primary goal in exercising is "toning" or "firming" their bodies, the information is presented here.

Firming your body is easier than working for strength, endurance, or size. You don't have to push it; however, more work makes more firmness. Just going running or doing aerobics classes, by themselves, may burn fat, so that you have better muscular definition, and they can work your leg muscles, but they won't firm your entire body. You need to work each area that you want to firm, through resistance exercise. The resistance can be your body weight, weight machines, or free weights.

How to Improve Your Different Aspects of Fitness

Cardiovascular Endurance (aerobic capacity). Long-duration, low-intensity, large-muscle activity like walking, running, skating, dancing, cross-country skiing, swimming. Comfortable intensity.

Anaerobic Capacity. Short-duration, high-intensity activity like sprints, whether on land, in the water swimming or finning, or on a bicycle. Alternate short, hard exertions with easy ones. Work hard enough to get out of breath, rest briefly, then sprint again.

Strength. Weight lifting. For general strengthening programs, carefully find the heaviest weight your can lift 8–12 times. For serious strength building, do 4–8 lifts (reps). Work up to three sets of repetitions. Take long rests between sets. Don't skip major muscle groups—train them all so you can avoid orthopedic problems from unequal strength ratios.

Muscular Endurance. Do continuous repetitions of lifts or motions, with light weight and no rest between repetitions. Vary to avoid overuse.

Power. Weight lifting, or other activity involving moving a heavy or light object (including yourself) quickly. Fast execution of each lift or motion. Long rests. Great care to avoid injury.

Size. Weight lifting: 4 sets of 12. Heavy to moderate weight. Lift slowly. Short rests between sets. Exercise and eat low fat so muscles can't hide beneath fat stored under your skin.

Firmness. Regularly lift a comfortable weight a comfortable amount of times, for example 10 repetitions, building up to 1–3 sets. Work each area that you want to firm.

Flexibility. Stretch enough to move freely through the range of motion you need for activities, but don't force your joints into such looseness that they no longer work properly. Do regular comfortable stretching exercises. After each stretch, stretch in the opposite direction.

Can You Have It All?

To improve at specific sports or activities, you need to develop the systems used in that particular activity. For your health, work on all of your different aspects of fitness, rather than concentrating on any particular one and neglecting the others.

Do safe and sane weight lifting to develop strength, endurance, and power. Regularly walk, jog, cycle, swim, and dance to develop cardiovascular endurance.

Do regular stretching to develop healthful range of motion and reduce injury potential.

Check with your physician before starting any program. Get instruction and start easy, even too easy in the initial weeks of a new program. Get the feel of it first. Then, and this is important, get to like it. Progressively work up. Exercise does not have to hurt to be effective. If anything hurts, stop, and find out why. You can have gain without pain. And you can have it all.

4

What Does "Aerobic" Really Mean?

A friend of mine runs marathons. He always talks about this runner's high. But he has to go twenty-six miles for it. That's why I smoke and drink.
I get the same feeling from a flight of stairs.

—Larry Miller

Quiz

When are you most aerobic?

a. Sitting in a chair
b. Doing 50 sit-ups
c. Swimming 200 yards

The answer is (a). You have more aerobic than nonaerobic processes going on when you are sitting in a chair than either doing 50 sit-ups or swimming 200 yards. To understand why, you need to know what "aerobic" *really* means and how it relates to aerobic exercise.

A Quick Overview

"**A**erobic" is not just a type of exercise. It is a way your body makes energy, not only to do exercise, but to be alive at all. *Aero* is a Greek word meaning "air," and *bios* is another Greek word meaning "life." You need the oxygen in air all the time to manufacture the energy to stay alive, for all your body functions at rest, and for moving around. Using oxygen to make energy is called *aerobic metabolism.*

Although not an exact example, aerobic metabolism uses oxygen and the breakdown products of food the way a carburetor mixes oxygen with gasoline to combust into energy and combustion by-products. In your body, the combustion is much slower than in automobile engines. Also, unlike a car with only one energy manufacturing mode, you have three different energy-generating systems. Only one of these systems is aerobic, the one using oxygen. The other two are *an*aerobic. *An-* is a prefix meaning "without." Anaerobic processes make energy without oxygen. They use stored fuels and don't need oxygen.

You use your aerobic system just about all the time—sleeping, sitting in a chair, right now while reading. That's why you breathe just about all the time. It's when you begin physical activity that you need the boost from your two *an*aerobic systems as well. Your three systems contribute in different proportions during different length and intensity activities. That means that some activities use more aerobic than anaerobic processes, and so are called *aerobic exercises,* and other activities use more anaerobic processes, and so are not aerobic exercises. But all three of your systems work to do the same thing— to make an energy-giving molecule called ATP.

Aerobic Metabolism Is Not the Same as Aerobic Exercise

Your body makes energy to stay alive using three systems: one is aerobic, the other two are anaerobic (not aerobic). You use all three in different amounts, depending on what you are doing. You need your aerobic system all the time. You are using aerobic processes right now reading this, and even when you sleep.

You need a boost from your two nonaerobic systems when you exercise. When an exercise uses the aerobic system the most and also gives you cardiovascular benefits, the exercise gets to be called *aerobic exercise* but the term is often misused.

Your Universal Energy Molecule

A special body molecule called ATP is the universal energy molecule. ATP fuels the activity and life processes of all living things, from bacteria, to plants, to bats, to you.

ATP is short for *a*denosine *tri*phosphate. It's a *tri*phosphate because it has three phosphates. The third phosphate is held on with a lot of energy (a high-energy bond). Breaking off the third phosphate releases that energy. Think of ATP like one of those toy spring-snakes in a can. When you undo the latch, the snake springs out all over. The latch is the high-energy bond—just a little thing, but holding back much energy. When your body needs energy, it uses a bit of water and an enzyme to undo the latch of ATP, and Zing! Out springs energy. You have billions and billions of ATP molecules doing this all the time. Zing! Zing!

Figure 4.1. You get energy from millions of molecules of ATP by breaking their high-energy bond. You store a little ATP in your body, and make the rest using oxygen and the foods you eat.

All three of your energy systems (two anaerobic and one aerobic) work toward the same final common event—to make ATP. Your aerobic, oxygen-using system makes large quantities of ATP from fat, carbohydrate, and sometimes protein. It can make lots of ATP for long periods of time. That's a good thing—you need to fuel your body processes even when you are asleep. But your aerobic system just can't make all that ATP very fast.

Sometimes you begin an activity so quickly and intensely, that you can't supply your body with enough oxygen fast enough. So the first few seconds are fueled by your first anaerobic system of stored ATP. But you don't have much stored ATP, and you run out quickly. If you continue your activity, your body has to change over to your second system, also *an*aerobic, where you make ATP by breaking down glucose and another carbohydrate called glycogen that you store in your muscles and liver. This second system is also limited in how much ATP it can make. After several more minutes of continued activity, your third system, the aerobic energy system, begins to contribute more and more to the energy needs of your cells.

If you are exercising very hard, your body can't make the switch back to aerobic metabolism. Your aerobic system just can't work quickly enough to make the energy you need to do your exercise. Without aerobic metabolism, you have to continue using the quick-and-ready glucose and glycogen. A problem with that is you can't make much ATP that way so you get tired. Another problem is that without aerobic metabolism, your body can't remove lactic acid and other products that build up during *an*aerobic metabolism (more on this in a bit). So you feel a burning sensation. All of this forces you to slow to a pace that can be supplied with ATP energy aerobically. If you won't slow down, you are soon halted in your tracks, gasping and burning—anaerobic. In short, the harder and faster you work (or the more it hurts), the more anaerobic. The steadier, or more relatively comfortable the pace, the more oxygen, and the more aerobic.

Although people often equate hard exercise with aerobic exercise, the harder and faster you work, the more *an*aerobic processes you use. With a more relatively comfortable pace, you can use more oxygen and be more *aerobic*.
The better in shape you are, the harder you can work and still be comfortable and aerobic.

A Closer Look at Your Three Energy Systems

You use your three energy systems for different intensity and duration activities ranging on a continuum from quick power, to speed and strength, to long endurance. Here's a closer, but still simplified look.

	System 1	System 2	System 3
System Name	ATP-CP	Glycolysis	Oxidative-Aerobic
Type	Anaerobic	Anaerobic	Aerobic
Method	Stored ATP	Makes ATP from stored glucose and glycogen.	Makes ATP from carbohydrates, fats, and sometimes protein.
Uses Oxygen?	No	No	Yes
Duration	Very short—seconds	Short to medium—minutes	Long—hours
Intensity of activity	Very high	High to medium	Medium to low

System 1. ATP-CP

The original earth atmosphere was oxygen-free. The first living things made energy using only anaerobic processes. Several kinds of your cells, including muscle fibers, retain that anaerobic ability. Nerve cells can't work anaerobically, so they are sensitive to oxygen shortages. But muscle cells work both aerobically and anaerobically, so have a great capacity to vary metabolic rate—more than any other body system.

Extremely brief, high-intensity bursts of activity lasting less than about 10 seconds are anaerobic and use stored ATP in your muscles to give you immediate energy. This is the realm of power movements like opening a window, football sprints, lifting a suitcase or grocery bag, putting the shot, jumping for a tennis or basket ball, and kicking and punching in martial arts.

ATP stores energy until you need it. Biological energy is measured in calories. One mole of ATP can break apart to give you about 7–12 calories of energy to spend as you like (a mole is a chemical measurement of an awful lot of molecules—see the glossary). ATP gives you energy by breaking off its third phosphate. But then what happens to it? You still need to make energy, and without the third phosphate, adenosine triphosphate becomes only adenosine *di*phosphate, ADP, with just two phosphates. The low-energy bond of the second phosphate is as much use to you as a nearly run-out battery. You need to recharge it.

As rapidly as you break up ATP for energy using this system, another stored molecule called creatinine phosphate (CP) puts it back together. CP sits around in your muscles until you need it to give up one of its phosphates. CP sticks one of its phosphate on ADP to make ATP again. Because ATP and CP work together, the ATP system is also called the ATP-CP system, or phosphagen system. But now, how can you make more CP?

Your supply of CP is limited. When you are doing intense exercise and run low on CP, you must slow down enough to be aerobic again, using oxygen. Then oxygen helps make and replenish your ATP and CP stores, a process taking only a few minutes. The energy repayment comes from the calories in your next meal. Being in shape with good aerobic ability increases the rebuilding of anaerobic energy stores, aiding the anaerobic recovery process.

How to Improve Your Anaerobic Capacity. You need anaerobic training like sprint swimming to increase the enzymes that are part of the ATP-CP cycle. Eating these enzymes to increase performance won't work, no matter what the health food claims tell you. All enzymes are proteins and are destroyed by digestion if eaten. That's the job of digestion. They won't automatically reassemble back into enzymes on the other side of the intestinal wall (Chapter 14, "Nutrition Myths"). Only power and speed-specific exercise, and plenty of it, builds this system.

System 2. Anaerobic Glycolysis

When you continue activity past the point where your CP stores run low, your cells switch to energy system 2. This system breaks down glucose to make ATP. Breaking down glucose is called glycolysis (*lysis* means "breaking down"), pronounced gly-COL-ih-sis. This system needs no oxygen, so this process is alternately called *anaerobic glycolysis*.

Anaerobic glycolysis can make ATP quickly, just not very much of it. For comparison, glycolysis can make about 2 molecules of ATP for each molecule of glucose, while your aerobic system can make 36

ATPs. (Actually, glycolysis makes 4 molecules of ATP, but uses 2 ATPs to do it. Everything takes energy.)

When Do You Use Glycolysis? Glycolysis enables you to do longer activities than those using your ATP-CP system, but not as long as with aerobic energy-making processes. Since glycolysis can make ATP quickly, it allows more intense activity that aerobic processes. This is the strength and speed domain. Efforts of 1–3 minutes, like a 400-meter run, a 100-meter swim, and climbing a hill carrying a load, rely heavily on anaerobic glycolysis. Since this system is anaerobic, you can do many of these activities holding your breath, like swimming underwater. The extent of glucose and glycogen use depends whether your exercise is continuous and of long duration, or intermittent-exhaustive, and varies greatly with intensity. Typical recreational activities usually fall in a middle ground.

Glycolysis and the Food You Eat. Only carbohydrate, not protein or fat, can be turned into energy without oxygen. Your body can store a fair amount of glucose by chaining glucose molecules together into molecules called glycogen, which you store mainly in your muscles and liver. When you need more glucose for glycolysis, your body just breaks apart the glycogen. Glycogen is broken down to glucose in all cells, but this process is most active in muscle and red blood cells.

Restoring your muscle and liver glycogen stores after hard exercise depends on how much carbohydrate you eat, and how soon after activity you start eating. The optimum time for restocking is in the first 30 minutes after exercise, and the second restocking "window" is in the next 2 hours or so. If you don't eat much carbohydrate in this time period, you won't have as much glycogen, even as long as 5 days later, than you would have if you ate right away.

You can increase your muscle glycogen stores by regularly eating carbohydrates, particularly right after exercising. You also increase your stores over time by exercising enough to convince your muscles they have a reason to store more.

Remember that everything takes energy. It take ATP molecules to put glycogen molecules back together in your body so you can store them. The energy your body needs to do the restocking comes from ATP made by your aerobic system from oxygen and the food you eat. Remember, the aerobic system is the one that has to work all the time to supply the energy so you can breathe, pump blood, digest, and do all the things your body needs to do to stay alive.

Figure 4.2. How much glycogen energy you can store for your next activity depends on how soon after exercising you start eating and how much carbohydrate you eat.

What (Really) Is "Go for the Burn"? Breaking down glucose to make ATP takes 12 steps. The end product of glycolysis is pyruvate (or pyruvic acid). After pyruvate forms, it can go two ways. Without enough oxygen to carry off the hydrogen ions that form when you are working anaerobically, they stick onto the pyruvate, making it into lactate (or lactic acid). All the acid products building up produce a burning feeling. "Go for the burn" indicates you are *an*aerobic. It's not beneficial to your cardiovascular system; it's just waste products like lactic acid and extra hydrogen ions making your body acid-y, and stimulating your pain receptors to say "owww."

If you lower your intensity to where the available oxygen can supply your needs, then the oxygen can turn the lactic acid back to pyruvate by carrying off the hydrogen ions and combining with them to form water. The pyruvate becomes available for your last, and third system—your aerobic system.

"Go for the burn" is a sure signal that you are working
above your aerobic capacity. It means that you are
not aerobic.
When you are aerobic, the oxygen you breathe makes
lactic acid into pyruvate, which you can use for energy.
When you are not working aerobically, the lactic acid
builds up and stimulates your pain receptors.

Figure 4.3. When you break down stored sugar to make energy while working very hard (anaerobically), the process stops with lactic acid because there is not enough oxygen for how hard you are working. When you work aerobically, the lactic acid doesn't build up but can turn into pyruvate, which you use for more energy.

System 3. Aerobic—Oxidative Metabolism

When the duration of your activity is long, and intensity is low enough to be met without the anaerobic systems, your body signals your cells to begin the gradual change back to your aerobic system. Endurance events are primarily aerobic, and use oxygen (oxidative metabolism) to produce energy. Aerobic metabolism can make a great deal of ATP to carry through long events. Be happy you're not a lizard. Reptile and amphibian hearts and lungs are not developed enough to use aerobic (oxidative) metabolism. They rely on glycolysis. Lizards don't win many long races.

Aerobic metabolism uses stored carbohydrate, fat, and protein if necessary, in two interesting pathways to make ATP. The first pathway is the Krebs cycle, and the second is the electron transport chain. For more detail on these pathways, see the glossary. You make most of your ATP in the electron transport chain. The electron transport chain takes the hydrogen ions formed in the energy-making process and, by combining them with oxygen, makes lots of ATP instead of allowing the ions to stick onto pyruvate. The extra ions turn pyruvate into the burning lactate. With lactate, you can't get into the Krebs cycle, so you lose a large portion of your ATP production opportunities. Having oxygen makes the difference between stopping your energy-making processes with lactate (while you gasp and rub burning limbs) or restoring lactate to pyruvate, so the pyruvate can enter into aerobic energy-making processes.

The Difference Between Aerobic Metabolism and Aerobic Exercise

Your aerobic metabolism goes on all day and night, even when you're sitting around or sleeping, making a distinction between aerobic metabolism and aerobic exercise. Not everything that predominantly uses your aerobic system is aerobic exercise. What does "aerobic exercise" mean in light of the fact that you are aerobic even when you are sleeping?

The word "aerobic" describing a type of exercise was coined by Dr. Kenneth Cooper, "Father of Aerobics." The intensity must be high enough to give a cardiovascular training effect, or it is not aerobic exercise. The intensity must not be so high that you are primarily using your nonaerobic systems, making you out of breath or with burning muscles.

What About Walking?

It's true that slow walking mostly uses your aerobic system. It does not invoke much of your *an*aerobic systems because it is such low intensity. In this case, energy is supplied aerobically but it is not aerobic exercise. Faster walking may qualify as aerobic exercise depending how high you raise your heart rate and how long you walk. Walk so that you feel you are moderately exerting yourself for at least 10–20 minutes a few times each week to start gaining health benefits. Walk longer and harder, and add other forms of exercise, for fitness benefits.

What About Running, Swimming, and Biking?

Nothing is very aerobic if you do it so fast that you are out of breath and have to stop. Then you are exercising primarily *an*aerobically. That does not mean that it is bad, just that it will not give you cardiovascular (aerobic) training effects. To run or jog aerobically, try a pace that you can maintain for at least 10–20 minutes, and that feels comfortably hard. To swim or bike aerobically, do the same.

What About Football?

Short, high exercise intensities decrease the ability of your aerobic system to meet the demand of your activity. Football games may be long, but the actual exercise is extremely short. A few tens of yards and tackles at most. That does not mean that football is not a hard sport, just that it is not an aerobic one. It can be very nonaerobic precisely because it is so intense.

That introduces an interesting tidbit—a common sight is players clapping oxygen masks over their faces, believing it will help performance and recovery. The practice will not hurt them, but neither will it physically help. Football moves do not use oxygen for energy—the exercise bouts are just too short. Players use anaerobic fuel stored in their muscles. Oxygen supplementation only minimally increases blood levels since blood already carries almost all the oxygen it can hold. To put it technically, your oxygen saturation is usually around 97–98%. Plus, any small increase in blood oxygen saturation with bottled oxygen will be gone by the time players get back to the field and aligned in formation.

What About Sit-ups?

During short, anaerobic exercises you use stored ATP, CP, and glycogen. That's why doing the 50 sit-ups mentioned at the beginning of this story is not aerobic, and is metabolically less aerobic than sitting in a chair, where all your processes are just about 100% aerobic. Swimming 200 yards is not long enough to switch back to primarily aerobic metabolism.

If you are out of breath and your heart is pounding, you are more anaerobic than aerobic. Although you are breathing in plenty of oxygen, your body can't deliver and process it fast enough. Lactic acid builds. When you exercise aerobically, oxygen changes lactic acid back to pyruvate, which can be used to make ATP.

What About "Fat-Burner Classes"?

A popular fad exercise class is the "fat-burner." Fat-burner classes are lower intensity than regular exercise classes, yet advertising for these classes states that participants burn more fat. The reasoning given is that during high-intensity exercise, glycogen is the primary fuel, but with lower intensity activity, more fat is used as a primary fuel. A little knowledge of "aerobic metabolism" seems to be a dangerous thing.

Fewer total calories are burned in these classes than in more vigor-

Figure 4.4. You have three energy systems—ATP-CP, glycolysis, and aerobic. Each contributes in different amounts during different intensities and durations of exercise.

ous classes, because the intensity is lower. Even though fat would supply a greater percentage of the energy in a low-intensity class, not as much in total would be mobilized over the same period of time. High-intensity activities, done for the same period of time, burn more total fat and calories.

That does not mean that overweight beginning exercisers should start with high-intensity exercises. Prolonged low-intensity exercise is a safer start for a weight loss program. Even regular exercise of only 50% of your maximum ability helps reduce risk of high blood pressure, diabetes, and carviovascular disease, if it is regular.

Eating for Aerobic Exercise

Your body's preferred fuel for aerobic metabolism is fat. That does not mean you have to eat it, but that your body likes to use it from its stores. A trained endurance athlete's body will begin the change to fat-burning from glycolysis sooner than an out-of-shape person's body can. The in-shape body wants to preserve muscle carbohydrate stores as long as possible, because more carbohydrate allows exercise to continue longer. Preferentially using fat instead of glycogen is called glycogen sparing, and is a training adaptation that delays fatigue.

It is popular to market foods that "give you energy." Since the main energy fuel for aerobic exercise is fat, will just eating lots of fat give you energy for aerobic exercise? Eating an oxidative fuel like fat isn't the way to increase your aerobic ability. You need aerobic practice, like regularly swimming long laps. *See* the previous chapter, "Improving Your Fitness," for more on how to get in shape, and Chapters 14, "Nutrition Myths," and 17, "Ergogenic Aids" in Part II, for more on foods that do and don't help your physical abilities.

An Aerobic and Anaerobic Bike Ride

Now you know enough to follow the three simplified metabolic pathways through a sample physical activity—a bike ride.

You're sitting quietly, oxidatively aerobic. You decide to go out for a bike ride, stand up, and walk over to get your bike, with the help of some ATP-CP stored in your legs.

You lift your bike in another burst of ATP-CP, and carry it out the door and down the steps, rapidly shifting to anaerobic glycolysis.

You catch your breath and begin your ride, first an easy warm-up, then up a nearby hill. As you pick up the pace, your bodily processes speed up to manufacture more ATP for energy. You breathe faster to take in more oxygen to help make that ATP. But there's a limit to how fast your body can deliver oxygen to your cells and how fast your cells can process oxygen in oxidative energy production. In your uphill ride, your energy demand exceeds the oxidative supply. Your cells rapidly switch to a mostly anaerobic glycolytic system. You begin to pant. Had you regularly worked out and gotten in better shape, the energy demand would be within range of your aerobic system. You would now be comfortably supplying your leg muscles with oxidatively stoked energy, not likely to run low soon.

But your cells are switching to your energy production processes that don't need oxygen. These processes can make energy for only short periods of time. Without enough oxygen to carry off extra hydrogen ions that attach to the pyruvate that forms from anaerobic metabolism, the pyruvate becomes lactic acid. Hydrogen ions accumulate, dropping your pH to the acid. Your legs burn.

The terrain changes and the hill levels off. You drop intensity and slow your pedaling. After several more deep breaths you "pay back" your debt to your anaerobic system, and allow oxygen to turn lactic acid back into pyruvate. You settle into a comfortable aerobic pace. After 10 or so minutes of continuous pedaling you are about 50% aerobic and 50% glycolytic anaerobic. After another 10 to 20 minutes of exploring, the aerobic percentage might have risen to about 60–70%

or so. If your fitness level is high, it can climb higher, a response of a well-trained body to help spare muscle glycogen and delay fatigue.

You reach the halfway point, turn around, and pedal back, now mostly aerobic. You reach the hill, and enjoy the effortless coast downhill. Your energy needs are still supplied aerobically, even more than during your uphill and level-terrain ride, although you are now doing almost no exercise. During the aerobic portion of your ride, your body has been busy replenishing much of your stored muscle CP for your ATP-CP system, but not glycogen. For restocking glycogen, you need to eat and drink. Oop! You went too far downhill and missed the turnoff. You turn around and pedal back uphill, with a rush of ATP-CP. Seconds later shifting to primarily anaerobic glycolysis, but there's not as much glycogen stored as before. These few minutes seem much harder than the first strong pedals at the start of your ride. There's your street, and then the steps. Up the steps in another ATP-intensive effort.

You put your bike down and take off your jacket using all three systems. Sitting quietly after your ride, you are primarily running on aerobic metabolism again. You get a snack of bagels and fruit to begin restocking muscle and liver glycogen. The phone rings. You would jump up but your anaerobic fuel stores are low and you are tired. It's been a fun day of exercise.

5

What Does "Warm-Up" Really Mean?

Now King David was old and stricken in years; and they covered him with clothes, but he got no heat. Wherefore his servants said unto him, Let there be sought for my lord the King a young virgin: and let her stand before the King, and let her cherish him, and let her lie in thy bosom, that the lord the King may get heat.

—I Kings 1:1–2

What Is a Warm-up?

Getting warmed up for exercise doesn't mean stretching or deep breathing. Even some common activities done for warm-ups in exercise classes are not warm-ups.

"Warm-up" means doing enough muscular work to raise your body temperature several degrees. People usually call just about any preparatory activity a warm-up, but the term literally means to get warmer.

You are like an automobile engine that heats up with use. Not all the fuel you put into your car goes to move the car. Most of the fuel energy to move the engine parts is lost as heat. In you, about 75% of all the energy you use for making your heart beat, for digestion, and every other body process, turns into heat, too. Human energy inefficiency works in your favor to heat you to 98.6° Fahrenheit (37°C) at rest. That's good. If it didn't, your chemical processes wouldn't go as quickly and you wouldn't be able to move around as easily. Muscular work using your large muscles converts even more mechanical energy into heat, raising your temperature even further.

"Warm-up" is not synonymous with any old preparation
for exercise. It specifically means to raise your body
temperature, making exercise safer.

What Is Not a Warm-up?

You won't raise your body temperature with deep breathing, arm
waving, or small muscle activity. Many exercise classes start by having
you rise up and down on your toes, supposedly to warm up your
calves. Or alternately bending and straightening your elbows. Or
worse yet, with stretching. These are not warm-up activities. Your
biceps and calf muscles are too small to contribute enough heat to
warm your body. Starting out with small muscle activities will only
poop you out before you can start some real exercise. Stretching
doesn't warm you—there is not enough large muscle movement going
on. Moreover, stretching while you are still cold can microtear and
weaken your muscle fibers. People injure themselves over time with
six main stretching mistakes. The first is not waiting until after you are
warmed up before stretching. Read more about stretching in Chapter 6,
"Stretching and the Six Great Stretching Mistakes."

Stretching is not a warm-up. You need to warm up first
using continuous, large muscle exercises, before
stretching. Stretching before you are warmed up can injure
you in several ways.

Why Warm Up?

Warming up changes your body in several ways that make exercise
orthopedically safer, and lessen your chance of overdoing things with
your heart. By raising your resting body temperature, your muscles
become more pliable, more injury resistant, and can work faster.
Warmed-up muscles can stretch more, and endure more force without
tearing. Increased body temperature improves diffusion of oxygen,
carbon dioxide, and metabolites to and from tissues. Blood viscosity

lessens and blood vessels widen, slightly reducing resistance to blood flow in muscles including the heart. Abruptly beginning intense activity without adequate warm-up can leave you without enough blood and oxygen to your heart. In a study of men with chest pain accompanying exercise because of narrowed heart blood vessels, warming up increased the length of time they could walk before onset of chest pain.

Benefits of Warm-up

- Muscles can stretch farther without tearing.
- Muscles become more injury resistant.
- Muscles can work faster.
- Blood viscosity lessens.
- Needed chemical reactions in your body speed up.
- Your blood vessels widen, reducing resistance to blood flow.
- Blood and oxygen can get into your heart and muscles more easily.
- Carbon dioxide and waste products can get out of your tissues more easily.

How Does a Warm-up Work?

Your body's chemical processes are sensitive to small temperature increases. The enzyme reactions in your cells that produce energy and control body functions speed up proportionally as your body temperature rises. A 10° C rise would double the rate of enzyme reactions. This is called the Q_{10} Effect. Of course, your internal temperature could never change 10° without severe health consequences. But the few degrees that a warm-up raises your temperature uses the Q_{10} Effect to boost your athletic performance.

Who Doesn't Need a Warm-up?

You won't benefit by warm-up exercises if you're a lizard. Lizards are cold-blooded, meaning they can't change body temperature on their own. They have to lie in the sun before they're hot to trot. Their internal temperature changes as their environment changes so they are called *poikilotherms* (POY-kill-oh-thurms), which means "variable temperature." Warm blooded beasties like us maintain remarkably constant internal temperature at rest so we are called *homeotherms* (HOME-ee-oh-thurms), a word meaning "same temperature."

Like lizards, scuba divers are another group who may not benefit by warm-up activities, but for different reasons. Warmer body temperature allows more nitrogen to get in and out of you. Lower temperature inhibits nitrogen uptake and elimination. Studies found that divers who spent their entire dives cold were less likely to get decompression sickness. But a diver starting a dive warm would absorb more nitrogen. If that diver then chilled, which is common during a dive, eliminating that additional nitrogen slows, increasing decompression sickness risk.

Other activities benefit from warm-up. The more strenuous the activity, or the more range of motion you need, the more you need a warm-up. Even a not-very-strenuous activity like golf needs a good range of motion of your back, shoulders, and hips, making warm-up important.

How Do You Know When You're Warmed Up?

You're warm when you break a sweat. It takes 5–10 minutes of exercise to increase muscle temperature so give your warm-up at least that long.

Important Points for Warm-ups

- Start with large muscle exercises that move your upper legs and hips.
- Gradually increase the tempo.
- If anything hurts or doesn't want to move where you're moving, slow down.
- Spend 5–10 minutes to warm up.
- Break a sweat.
- Put off stretching until you're sweating.
- Don't overdo.
- Have fun so that you'll look forward to the next time.

Here's What to Do

You can warm up for exercise in three ways:

1. Active direct warm-up
2. Active indirect warm-up
3. Passive warm-up

An active direct warm-up is the same activity as the actual exercise but at a lower intensity. For example, fast walking warms you for jogging. Slow jogging warms you for running. Slow cycling warms you for faster cycling. Slow swimming is a good warm-up for pool training.

An active indirect warm-up uses any large muscle activity such as pedaling a bicycle. In an exercise class, look for rhythmic leg motions that use the large muscles of the leg, not small muscle activity such as arm movements and heel raises.

For active warm-ups, start with large muscle exercises that move upper legs and hips. Large muscle activity converts more mechanical energy into heat. Start off easy then gradually increase the work. If anything hurts or doesn't want to move where you're moving, slow down.

For a passive warm-up, get in a sauna, steam, or conventional hot bath. Your body temperature rises with passive warm-up, although passive warm-up lacks the circulatory benefits of active exercise. That's not to say passive warm-up isn't useful. Hot steamy showers give people with arthritis or other injuries the head start on muscle heat they need to reduce pain and increase range of movement enough to start exercising actively. Just drink extra water to avoid dehydration.

Spend 5–10 minutes warming up, and continue until you break a sweat. Don't stretch until after you're sweating. Most important, have fun so that you'll look forward to the next time.

6

Stretching and the Six Great Stretching Mistakes

One learns to itch where one can scratch.

—Ernest Bramah

Have you ever started to fall asleep while sitting up in a chair? You struggled to stay awake. When you lost the battle, your head slumped forward only to suddenly jerk back up again. Pulling your head back up was not a voluntary move. It was a reflex that resulted from stretches and bounces. This chapter will tell you more about it, and how that relates to stretching right.

This chapter also covers the Six Great Stretching Mistakes. Although flexibility can reduce injuries, stretching incorrectly can produce them. Bouncing on stretches increases flexibility but can cause injuries. Stretching isn't a warm-up. You need flexibility but you also have a few bodily structures you should not stretch at all.

Benefits of Stretching

With good flexibility, you may suffer fewer injuries to your muscles and the tough fibrous structures called tendons that attach your muscles to your bones. Although not all studies support the conclusion of fewer injuries, the reasoning has good basis. If a muscle is tight, its inflexibility limits the range it can achieve. If you move in a way that surpasses that range, you may strain or tear the muscle and its connecting tendons. A tight-jointed person may have a greater tendency for muscle pulls and strains.

Several body areas appear susceptible to injury from poor flexibility. The range of motion required to strain tight low back muscles is quite small, accounting for many painful backs after a day of recreational fun. Your Achilles tendon at the back of your lower leg attaches your calf muscle to your heel. Tight calf muscles and Achilles tendons sometimes lead to tendonitis, knee pain, and foot pain, if you don't wind up with an outright tear. Another susceptible area is the triple set of muscles called the hamstrings, that connect the back of your hip to your leg. Tight hamstrings are prone to "pulls." Tight hamstrings may be a common contributor to low back pain because they change the normal angle of the hip and low back.

The muscles that connect the front of your hip to your leg are called hip flexors. Hip flexors bend your leg forward (flex it) at the hip. Tight hip flexors, common in people who sit a lot, change the normal angle of the hip and low back, adding a large share of low back pain, and limit the range of hip and leg motion needed for efficient walking, running, and even reaching overhead.

Tight hip and leg muscles are a major contributor to low back pain. When these muscles are tight, common in people who sit a lot, it changes the normal angle of the hip and low back, and inhibits normal walking and running. Tight hip muscles even prevent normal torso motion when reaching overhead, contributing to shoulder pain.

Tight hip flexors are an amazing hidden cause of shoulder pain. When you reach overhead, your hip must be flexible enough to let your upper body lean back from the hip. When hip motion is limited by tightness, your shoulder has to overcompensate when reaching overhead, by bending and rotating too far back. The repetitive strain on the shoulder during weight lifting, tennis, football, and any overhead activity, even reaching overhead shelves, can produce shoulder pain that is hard to rehab if you do not also stretch the tight hips that are causing the malalignment in the first place.

Figure 6.1. A little lack of flexibility can contribute to a lot of problems. Tight hip muscles change the normal angle of your hip and low back, and limit the range of motion you need for normal walking, running, and even reaching overhead.

The Six Great Stretching Mistakes

Regular stretching has several health benefits. Your muscles can attain a greater length before reaching the point required to tear them. Your joints can line up properly, avoiding wear and tear. When muscles are too tight, unequal tensions develop in joints, often leading to pain and injury. So what could be bad about stretching for flexibility? Here are six common mistakes.

1. Stretching Before Warm-up

Stretching cold muscles is one way to injure yourself. At cooler muscle temperatures it takes less force and stretch to tear the muscle fibers. "Warming up" literally means increasing your body temperature. Activities that warm you enough to safely begin exercise are large muscle exercises like pedaling a bicycle or slow jogging. Stretching doesn't raise your body temperature so it's not a warm-up. Wait to stretch until *after* you warm up. When you've exercised enough to get sweaty, you're warmed up enough to stretch. *See* Chapter 5 for more on warm-ups.

- Stretching is not a warm-up.
- Stretching before warming up can lead to muscle tears, cramps, and other injuries.
- Warm up at least 5–10 minutes before stretching.
- You're warmed up when you begin to break a sweat.

2. Stretching Ligaments, Not Muscles

Ligaments are fibrous bands that hold your bones together so you don't rattle around. Ligaments normally are not supposed to stretch much. They retain their length, within a range, to hold your bones in position so the bones glide past each other along anatomically healthy paths.

Your joints need to be flexible, but not too loose either. When injury or chronic improper stretching forces ligaments to lengthen, they do not readily go back to their former length. Technically speaking they are *plastic* but not *elastic*. Stretched ligaments hang shapelessly loose like worn-out underwear waistbands. What's so bad about that? A couple of things.

Stretched ligaments don't hold your bones in line, allowing them to rub and grind at unhealthy angles. The friction contributes to degenerative changes over time and all the pain and disability that accompanies it. Ligament laxity predisposes to sprains and dislocations. For example, too much looseness on the sides of your ankle increases your chance of ankle sprains. Lax shoulder capsules may slip out of place from forces that healthier joint capsules tolerate. People with overly lax joints need strengthening exercises for the supporting musculature, to offset the potential for injury.

Everyone has different amounts of natural ligament looseness. Men generally have less natural flexibility than women, but can attain healthy flexibility with regular stretching. Some people have too much flexibility. Extreme ligament laxity is a common problem among dancers, and sometimes swimmers who overdo shoulder stretching. Although dancers need extreme flexibility for their art, and swimmers get better reach and range, it is not always healthy for them. With the increasing popularity of exercise classes, ligament damage is becoming common in the general population from improper stretching instruction. These people need strengthening programs to compensate for their acquired structural problem and the damage that can result.

There are several things you can do to avoid stretching ligaments when you really want to stretch muscles. Two are most important:

1. Keep the limb you're stretching in line with the joint. Several well-known stretches hold the joint at an angle that puts too much weight and pressure on ligaments. The "hurdler's stretch" is a major example. It twists your knee sideways. Instead, keep the nonstretched leg in front of you with your foot on the floor. Forcing your arms high up behind you strains the front, and weakest part, of your shoulder capsule. There's no need to stretch your arms like that.
2. Avoid constant pressure on joints over extended periods of time. An example is continuously sitting with a rounded back. Slouching overstretches the long ligament running up and down the back of your spine called the posterior longitudinal ligament. A chronically overstretched posterior longitudinal ligament weakens your back, and can lead to disc trouble (*See* Chapters 20 and 21, "Back and Neck Pain"). Habitually standing with your head forward stretches the back of your neck, with similar results. Squatting on your "haunches" pries knee ligaments apart, particularly if you have heavy legs. Continuous, long-term squatting damages the small discs of cartilaginous cushion in your knees, called meniscus. The bad knees of professional baseball catchers come from chronic squatting.

- Ligaments normally are not supposed to stretch much.
- Stretched ligaments don't hold your bones in line, allowing them to rub and grind at unhealthy angles.
- Avoid putting weight and pressure on ligaments, such as in the "hurdler's stretch" and pulling your arms high up behind you.
- Avoid constant pressure on joints over extended periods of time, such as slouching, which weakens muscles and joints, and pressures the discs.

3. Putting More Weight on Joint Capsules Than They Can Stand

Your joints are places where your body crams many structures into little space. Because of that, it's easy to do things that squash, tear, and abrade your joints. Joint cartilage and ligaments have a poorer blood supply than other body parts. Low blood supply means slow repair that may not keep up with each small destructive incident. Some damaged joints never heal, forcing their owners into surgery. Damage usually occurs slowly without your knowing it is happening and can, over time, injure your joint to the same degree as can a single accident. Chronic mistreatment slowly thickens a joint with fibrous scar tissue. Scarring makes the capsule less mobile and more uncomfortable as small abuses gradually accelerate the normal wear and tear of aging.

Examples of well-known stretch-intensive activities that can damage your joints are squatting on your heels and duck walks, both of which force the knee joint open. Avoid neck manglers like the "plow"— lying with your legs in the air over your head and all your weight on your shoulders and neck.

A stretch that puts too much weight on your spine is bending over from a stand for toe touching, or worse—bouncing while bending over for toe touching. Stretches like that do more harm than good. You don't need them. To stretch your hamstrings without hurting your back, lie on your back, bend both knees, then leave one foot on the floor and straighten the other leg overhead. Most foolhardy of all is bent-over weight lifting like straight-legged dead lifting. *See* Chapters 20 and 21 on back pain.

- It's easy to squash, tear, abrade, and scar your joints when you put more weight on them than they were designed for.
- Examples of stretches that overweight a joint are the "plow," duck walk, standing toe touch, and straight-legged dead lift.
- Damage can occur slowly without your knowing it, and can injure your joints over time as much as from a single accident.

4. Unequal Stretching

It is common to overdo stretching in one direction without countering the stretch in the opposite direction of movement. An obvious example is dancers who stretch their legs outward without equal and opposite stretching inward. The outside of their legs gradually tightens and shortens, the inside loosens, until they walk like ducks. Later their hips and knees succumb to early wear.

Another easily recognized example is round-shouldered muscle men. They build up their chest without stretching it, which tightens and shortens it. Their back cannot counter the pull of their strong and shortened big chests. Their chests pull them into a round-shouldered posture. This posture can slowly cause back and neck pain. Sometimes the shortening is so extensive that it pulls on the shoulder where the upper arm attaches. The upper arm rotates so that their thumbs face inward, sometimes even backward, rather than forward.

Figure 6.2. It is common to stretch too much in one direction and not enough in the other. You may overstretch your back but not stretch your front, so that you become round-shouldered. Some people do this so much that their arms rotate inward. Or the inside and outside of your legs may be unequally tight, which allows them to turn in one direction more than the other. These postures can cause early wear and tear on your joints.

The most common example of unequal stretching is when ordinary people chronically round their back and hip all day long by sitting, standing, and walking with poor posture. The only stretching they do, if any, is more forward motion during toe touches, sit-ups, leg lifts, and chest exercises. Damage builds up gradually. The consequences of an overstretched back and a tight chest range from poor posture, pot belly, and shallow breathing, to back pain and disc injury. This is also the least recognized example. It is so common that it looks "normal."

After stretching in one direction, stretch the other way. (Check with your physician before any new exercises.) After each half hour or so of sitting get up and stretch backward. Or lie face down propped up on your elbows. When standing or sitting, keep your ear centered over your shoulder not in front or behind it to keep your neck from overstretch. *See* Chapters 21 and 22 on back pain, for more on this important issue.

Figure 6.3. An overstretched back and tight chest are so common that they look normal. The bent forward postures that result can lead to back pain and disc injury.

- Stretching in one direction without countering the stretch in the opposite direction can cause injury and make you stand and walk funny.
- Examples of unequal stretching are stretching forward for toe touches, chest exercises, and ab exercises, but never stretching backward. Round shoulders, poor posture, and back pain commonly result.

5. Bouncing

Bouncing forces your muscles to an unsafe length before your pain receptors have time to signal you not to do such a thing. Bouncing can increase your flexibility but at the cost of microinjuries, and is one of several reasons you sometimes get sore after exercise. Bouncing is called ballistic stretching. By contrast, slow stretches called static stretches are not usually associated with delayed-onset soreness, and may help relieve soreness after you've already overdone it. There is some debate whether static stretching ahead of time reduces the delayed soreness of too much exercise. *See* Chapter 10, "Just Overdo It."

Sense organs all over your body that pick up and send information about what's happening to your body are called proprioceptors. *Proprio* means "self," and the word root *ceptors* refers to "receiving information." Proprioceptors tell you about yourself. The most abundant proprioceptors in your body are structures called muscle spindles.

Spindles lie embedded in your muscles. Bouncing has an interesting effect on your muscles because of these muscle spindles. When you stretch a muscle quickly, the spindle stretches too, activating its sensory nerve. The sensory nerve carries a message to your spinal cord about how much and how fast your muscle stretched. Your nervous system sends a signal back down to tell your muscle not to stretch so much.

An example is maintaining balance. You make thousands of minor adjustments all day without thinking about it, while sitting, standing, and walking. If you lean forward, the spindles in your back and the back of your legs stretch. They signal your spine to send a return message to your muscles; not only to contract, but how much to contract. They pull you back to an upright position, but no further. The muscle stretch-contraction loop is called the myotatic reflex, or stretch reflex.

The sudden stretch of bouncing activates muscle spindles. Your spindles send a sensory message up your neural chain of command, triggering a motor message back down to contract the muscle. Bouncing again during the contract reflex forces the muscle to lengthen against the energy of its own contraction. Damage can occur in the structures that both stretch and resist the stretch.

Remember falling asleep in your chair at the beginning of this story? When the sudden stretch of your head bouncing forward activated neck muscle spindles, the message came back to contract your neck muscles just as suddenly, pulling your head back up again. Now you know it was your muscle spindles at work in a stretch reflex.

- Bouncing while stretching can increase your flexibility but can cause tiny (or large) muscle and joint pulls and tears.
- Bouncing sends your nervous system a signal to make the muscle contract, to protect it from tearing. So bouncing can sometimes make your muscle tighter.
- Hold your stretch about 30 seconds without bouncing.

6. Stretching Without Strengthening

Being highly flexible, by itself, does not make you a better person, or more fit. It can even create problems. A joint must be able to move, but not so much that it moves out of place, rubs adjacent structures, or jangles loosely during daily movement. It is important to keep the musculature surrounding your joints strong, to support your joints, and maintain joint movement in healthy directions and ranges.

- By itself, being flexible is not synonymous with being in good shape.
- Stretching a joint without exercising it to be strong may allow it to stretch too far.
- Combine strengthening exercises with your stretching exercises.

Protect Your Back During Stretching

- Don't overload your back during stretches.
- Do back stretches sitting or lying down.
- Keep the normal inward curve of your lower back.
- Avoid sitting with a rounded back and a forward head.
- Don't push or force back stretches and don't let anyone help you stretch by pushing or forcing.
- Stretch in both directions—if you stretch by leaning forward then stretch by leaning backward. Make an even arc with your back, rather than just "folding" at one easily moved joint.

Here's What to Do

Stretch Often

Reduce your injury potential by stretching often, because unlike strength gains from weight training, flexibility gains are easily lost.

Stretch Safely

Warm up enough to sweat before you stretch. Then slowly ease into your stretch, then hold. Don't bounce or you'll activate your myotatic stretch contraction loop. Microinjuries can result. Easy-Does-It is better for you than forcing. Forcing stimulates your spindle reflex to give your muscle a shrink, not a stretch.

Stretch Evenly

To avoid posture problems and back pain from unequal stretching, practice safe backs during stretching. Stretch your upper back, lower back, and hip in each natural direction. Don't overload your back. Substitute sitting and lying back stretches for standing-bent-over ones. Avoid sitting with a rounded back. Keep the normal inward curve of your lower back.

Points For Stretching

- Warm up before you stretch.
- Slowly ease into your stretch, then hold.
- Don't bounce.
- Easy does it. Stretch in a comfortable range, not forced to the point of pain.
- Stretch joints in each natural direction, not only in one.
- Don't stretch any joint in any unnatural position.
- Breathe normally while stretching; don't hold your breath.

7

Abdominal Muscles— Why You Need Good Ones, and How to Get Them

He was a man of an unbounded stomach.

—Katharine, in Shakespeare's
King Henry VIII, Act 4, scene 2

Your abdominal muscles have a busy schedule. When they're in good shape, they are among your main posture muscles. Abdominal muscles help keep your spine and hip bones at healthy angles for the postural control that avoids early wear and tear, and back pain. You use your "abs" to lift things, shout over distances, breathe during hard exercise, protect your internal organs, and assist childbirth. A little improvement to your abs can boost your overall quality of living.

Everyone benefits by building good abdominal muscles, but how? Two exercises popularly thought to benefit abs—sit-ups and leg lifts—don't work them as well as other exercises. They are also tough on your back. Why is that? What can you do instead? Why do strong abs help your back? What exercises flatten your abdomen and what if you don't like to go to a gym?

How Your Muscles Work

To understand how to improve your abdominal muscles, there are important things to know about muscles in general. All muscles originate on a bone, cross a joint, then attach to another bone on the other side of the joint. When a muscle contracts, it pulls on the bones to bend the joint it crosses. Your biceps muscle in front of your upper arm, for instance, contracts to bend your elbow. Muscle can only contract and pull. It cannot actively lengthen to push the bone away. To do that, another muscle on the opposite side of the bone contracts to pull the joint the other way. To straighten your elbow, other muscles called triceps in back of your arm contract.

How Your Abs Work

Your abdominal muscles connect your ribs to your hipbones. When your abs contract, they pull your ribs closer to your hips, moving your torso. By contrast, sit-ups and leg lifts move your body and legs closer together, principally using muscles that connect your back bones to your legs, moving your hip. More on this in a bit.

Your abs were named for their layout in your body. The abdominal muscle that runs straight down your front is your rectus abdominis, which in Latin means "the straight abdominal muscle." Your rectus abdominis starts where your ribs come together in the middle and runs straight down to the front of your pelvic bone.

The abs that orient diagonally across your trunk are your oblique abdominals. The obliques are interesting muscles. The outer set, called external obliques, originate at your sides and run diagonally down to your pelvic bone. If you put your fingertips in your pants pockets, your hands line up in the direction of the external oblique muscle fibers. When the external oblique fibers on the right side of your body contract, they pull your right side closer to the middle of your pelvic bone. In other words, you twist to the left. When you contract your left external oblique, you twist to the right. When you contract both, you bend forward.

Your internal obliques lie under your external obliques, in the opposite direction. Cross your arms over your abdomen. Your fingers assume the direction of the internal fibers. Your right internal oblique contracts to pull the middle of your ribs to the outside of your right hip, twisting you to the right. The left internal oblique twists you to the left in similar fashion. Yet another abdominal muscle, the transversus, helps compress the abdomen.

To summarize the action of your ab muscles:

- To twist to your right, you contract your left external oblique and right internal oblique.
- To twist to your left, you use your right external oblique and left internal.
- To bend forward, you use all abdominal muscles except the transversus.

Figure 7.1. Your rectus abdominis muscle runs from your ribs to the front of your pelvic bones. When this muscle is in good shape, it prevents your torso from swaying backward, like a guy wire between your ribs and pelvis.

Why Do Good Abs Help Your Back?

Of several theories relating abdominal muscles to back health, some are debated hotly. The following two are well substantiated.

Your rectus abdominis muscle is like a support strut in the front. Your obliques stabilize your torso from the sides. All together, they maintain slight tension all the time to prevent you from swaying backward while standing and sitting. People with weak abs can't maintain their posture to keep their vertebrae in healthy positions. Years of rubbing and straining at bad angles contributes to early wear and back pain.

Your oblique muscles attach into a fibrous sheath that connects to your back muscles. Strong obliques pull these back muscles to each side like a dynamic corset. By reinforcing the support structure for your back, good obliques reduce load and strain on your back muscles.

Why Don't Sit-ups and Leg Lifts Work Your Abs?

In the classic sit-up, you raise your trunk toward your leg by bending at the hip. Leg raises lift your legs closer to your trunk, also by bending at the hip. Bending the hip is called hip flexion. The muscles working during sit-ups or leg lifts are your hip flexors. They lie deeper than your abdominals, and they are mostly what you feel working when you do sit-ups and leg lifts.

Your main hip flexor muscle crosses your hip. Your abdominal muscles do not cross the hip, and so, are not used in hip flexion. If they were, you could work out your abdominals by the most frequent form of dynamic hip flexion—walking.

Why Can Sit-ups and Leg Lifts Hurt Your Back?

Sit-ups and leg lifts contribute to back pain in two ways. Two of your hip flexor muscles attach to your lower spine. Your spine was not built to withstand the constant yanking.

Figure 7.2. Sit-ups and leg lifts (including leg lifts in which you bicycle your legs) can contribute to back pain even if you are in good shape.

Another problem with sit-ups and leg lifts occurs when they shorten your hip flexor muscles. This shortening is common in people who sit a lot, and who overdo hip flexor exercise without stretching their hip flexors. Several problems can result:

- Short, tight hip flexors pull your pelvis forward. The shift in the normal tilt is one of several contributors to low back pain.
- Tight hip flexors yank on your back bones with every step you take.
- Tight hip flexor muscles can contribute, surprisingly, to shoulder injuries. Tight hip flexors do not allow full range of motion of your torso, so that when you try to reach overhead, your shoulder has to overrotate.
- Hip flexor muscles can sometimes be so tight that they prevent you from lying flat. They pull on the hip so much that the low back is pulled from the floor when the legs are stretched out. That is why many specialists recommend, for people who sleep on their back, to keep a small pillow under their knees to prevent back pain. With the knees bent up by the pillow, the tight hip flexors cannot pull the back into an arch. These people are especially in need of regular hip flexor stretches. (For more on back pain, *see* Chapters 20 and 21.)

These are better exercises for your abs without the risk sit-ups and leg lifts pose to your back. Unless you need extraordinary hip flexor strength for rugby, ballet, springboard diving, martial arts, or gymnastics, and are willing to take extra care to avoid back strain and do extra hip flexor stretches, stick with the exercises described below, for ab work.

"Ab-Only" Exercises Are Not Good

Abs create an important support structure for your lower torso and back, but they are not the entire support. Many people mistakenly do only abdominal muscle exercises, thinking it will make their backs injury free. There are two problems with this.

1. Without adding exercises that actively contract your back muscles, you will reach a point where your weaker back muscles can't counter the chronic muscle tension developed in front from

Figure 7.3. When the muscles in front of your hip are tight, that leg will come up, rather than lie flat, when you raise the other. Tight hip muscles can contribute to several posture and back pain problems.

your abs. The resulting forward pull encourages your body to slouch forward as your natural state—a poor posture that people are usually already very good at. This forward-slouching posture slowly puts unhealthy pressure on the vertebrae and nerves that exit the vertebrae. It pressures your discs to bulge out toward the back, and overstretches your back muscles. Keeping your back muscles, or any muscles, lengthened by poor posture weakens them.

2. Because your abs attach to your pelvic bone in front, too much muscle tension from abs, unbalanced by low-back muscles, pulls your pelvis into a tilt that adds to back pain.

You won't feel a problem right away. This kind of back injury takes time to develop, so have patience.

Not surprisingly, "ab-only" exercises contribute to back pain and poor posture.
Add exercises that contract your back muscles, called lumbar extension exercises, to balance the supporting muscles for your torso.

What Really Works Your Abs?

One approach to improving your abdomen is to go to a gym, but then neglect your abs the other 23 hours a day. It sometimes works. Another plan is to use your abs all day. Contract your abs tightly right now. Now let them bulge out completely loose. Somewhere between the two is a good tension to maintain for daily wear.

When you stand up, notice if your low back sways. If you do, add tension to your abs to lessen the curve a bit and bring you upright. If you slouch forward, lift up and back, and pull in your abdomen. Test your posture while standing with your back against a wall. No need to be a soldier, just see if your head, upper back, behind, calves, and heels all touch the wall at once. There should be a small space between your low back and the wall, but not a large space. When you sit, sit upright without slouching or rounding your back. Stand and sit well all the time and you'll exercise your abs without working out. *See* Chapters 20 and 21 on back pain and prevention.

Why kill yourself working out, but ignore your abs the
other 23 hours a day?
Stand and sit well all the time and you'll exercise your abs
without working out.

The most common ab exercise is trunk flexion, also called trunk curls, or crunches, pictured below.

Figure 7.4. Trunk flexion, also called trunk curls or "crunches," works your abdominal muscles. Contract or "curl" your torso forward, and do not move your legs. If you support your head with your hands, keep your neck in normal posture, not pulled forward which can overstretch your neck and add to bad posture over time. Alternatively, keep your hands on your chest.

Don't secure your feet under anything. That brings your hip flexors back into play. Lift your torso with your abdominal muscles, not your neck. Don't clasp your hands behind your head or neck. Don't throw yourself forward with your arms, that's cheating. To exercise your obliques, raise your elbow to your knee on the same side. Twisting to each opposite knee, as is commonly done, simultaneously flexes and rotates the spine, which is hard on it. The twisting move produces cosmetic results for your abs, but can be injurious over time.

There are several exercises to target the lower fibers of your abdominal muscles:

- To begin, lie on your back, with your feet on the floor. Feel where the small of your lower back arches slightly off the floor. Flatten that arch out by pushing your lower back into the floor, contracting your lower abdomen tightly. When you release, your back returns to a small arch. This is called the Pelvic Tilt and is a useful exercise to mobilize your low back and hip, learn the tilting motion of the hip and how it relates to your posture, and feel which muscles work to accomplish that.
- Lie on your back, bending at the hip, so that both your legs are straight up, extended above you. Contract your abdominal muscles, which curls your torso, to raise your hips from the floor. Don't bend your legs closer to your trunk—that's hip flexion, not abdominal work.

Tips for Crunches

If your neck hurts when doing crunches, you may be straining on each lift. Besides watching your form, and strengthening your neck, you can stop neck strain by pressing the back of your head into your hands, rather than yanking your head up with your hands. The pressing back activates muscles in the back of your neck. This activation quiets muscular activity in the front of your neck in an interesting action called *reciprocal inhibition.* That means that when one set of muscles works, the muscles that oppose them on the other side cannot work. It will stop the muscles in front of your neck from hurting.

To make an inexpensive "ab machine," just use a towel. Hold it between each hand, and use it to cradle your head and neck when you do your crunches. To make an inexpensive "ab machine *plus,*" use a small dumbbell instead of the towel, and press the back of your head against the bar.

Remember, the purpose of ab work is not to bend your neck farther forward. That posture is called slouching and is bad for your back and neck. It makes you look older. It's a shame that so many people practice exactly that every time they go to the gym. Keep your neck straight, don't yank or pull it forward. Ab work is supposed to make your life and your posture better, not bent over like an old tree.

A Much Neglected, Yet Great Ab Exercise

When you exercise a muscle, that muscle gets good at what you make it practice. That means that when you do crunches, you develop your ability to curl your torso forward and back and forward and back. Is that what you really wanted? Think a minute. When do you need to do that in a day? Chances are that you rarely do that, unless you're a professional Japanese greeter. Even for getting up from lying on your back, it's safer for your back not to sit up directly. Back specialists advise that you roll to one side first.

Your abs need to stay contracted at one length all day for you to sit, stand, walk, run, and carry packages properly. Holding a muscle in tension at just one length is called *isometric*. Your abs, like many of your other postural muscles, function normally in an isometric manner. When you use your abdominal muscles to maintain good posture, which is their main job, you hold them with enough tension that you do not stand with a swayback or fall over backwards. So exercise your abdominal muscles that way, too, to make them better at it. You can benefit by exercising your abs in the manner in which they normally work.

The ab exercises you see everywhere in gyms get you good at bowing forward and back, and forward and back. But your abs normally work isometrically—at one length so you can stand up without slouching, not by bowing your entire torso forward. So exercise your abs isometrically for postural control and normal function.

That means a radically different exercise than you commonly see in gyms and on exercise videos:

- Lie on your back with your knees bent, and feet on the floor. Keep the natural curve in your back without arching and without pressing your back hard into the floor. Hold your arms overhead a few inches above the floor. Feel your abs contract to hold your torso straight without allowing your back to arch up off the floor.

- When you can comfortably do this, add a small weight to your hands, making sure your low back does not arch. Your abdominal muscles work hard on this one. Holding the hand weight also works your latissimus dorsi muscles along the side of your back.

- Increase the weight slowly and safely as you improve your abs so that they can maintain your low back in good neutral posture.

- To increase the difficulty of this exercise as you progress, extend your legs, so that your knees are less bent. Keep your low back pressed against the floor.

- As long as you can safely progress the difficulty, work until you can properly do this isometric ab exercise, with hand weights, with your legs completely straight out on the floor, and your low back still in good neutral posture.

- You may also need to stretch your hip flexor muscles so that you can straighten your legs without arching your low back.

Important note: Anyone with cardiovascular disease and/or hypertension should not do sustained isometric contraction of their upper extremities such as this. Consult with your physician.

Figure 7.5. Your abs normally work isometrically—at one length—so you can stand, sit, and walk without arching. In this isometric ab exercise, you don't allow your back to arch, which contracts your abs in a way similar to how you need them in life. This is good for posture control and normal function.

How Much Ab Exercise Should You Do?

To gain strength, your muscles must contract at tensions close to their maximum, a concept called overloading. You need heavy resistance with few repetitions to overload a muscle. How heavy? A weight heavy enough that you can't lift or move it more than 8–12 times. Ab exercises are usually done using your own body weight as resistance. If you can only do about 10 repetitions of your ab exercise, then your body weight is enough by itself to increase your ab strength. If you can do more repetitions, then the resistance is too light, and you will increase endurance more than you increase strength.

- To increase strength, hold a small weight or lie on a slant board so that 8–12 repetitions is your limit.
- To gain endurance, do high repetitions with or without extra weight.
- Work up to 3 sets 3 times a week.

How Do You Flatten Your Abdomen?

No exercise selectively removes fat from any target body part. That myth is called "spot reducing." If spot reducing worked, people would have thin mouths from talking, and the repetitive act of chewing and swallowing lots of food would make your face thin.

Aerobic exercise burns fat. This fat comes from everywhere it is stored. That means to lose fat, including fat from your abdomen, you need to run, swim, bike, row, dance, skate, jog, ski, or walk. Ab exercises alone will not remove fat from your abdomen. That does not mean that resistance exercise does not have a place in weight control. Weight training builds muscle, which raises your metabolic rate. A higher rate means your body burns more calories every day.

Ab exercise helps compress your abdomen, and tone your abdominal muscles. Ab exercise is part of the work you need for the good posture that pulls your back and hips into better alignment, so that you don't stand with your abdomen sticking out. How ironic that many exercises mistakenly done in gyms tighten the hip and ignore the back so that you do just that.

How Do You Get a "Washboard"?

You have bands of fibrous tissue called fascia that run across your abdominal muscles at intervals. Doing good abdominal work will enlarge the muscles enough to poke through the facial bands, giving a "washboard" or "ripple" effect. You won't see that if body fat covers everything. The entire package of getting results consists of proper abdominal exercise, good posture, adequate carbohydrate and water in your diet to fuel good workouts, and reduced fat under your skin to produce a beautiful washboard abdomen.

8

What Exercises Do You Need to Be Fit?

I do not like work even when someone else does it.

—Mark Twain

What is fit? Does it mean just being healthy? Clearly, someone completely out of shape may not have a fun time during a hike or exercise class. Yet fitness is specific to the exercise you use to "get fit." Olympian shot putters may be fit to put the shot, but not for gymnastics or an aerobics class. Some people play tennis as their exercise for the week, but tennis won't get you fit for hiking or swimming, and it won't get all your body parts and systems fit. There are health benefits to the commonly heard exercise "prescription" of 3 times a week for 20 minutes, but you still may not be cardiovascularly "fit" enough to get you through a day without fatigue, or muscularly fit to get you through a day without back pain.

Chapter 2 explained the different aspects of fitness, and Chapter 3 covered how to improve each different aspect of fitness. Chapter 13 explains that you don't even need to go to the gym if your lifestyle involves lots of varied physical activities. So what exercises are good for you to get fit? This chapter covers the different types of exercise to improve the different aspects of fitness, to improve your different body parts, and to avoid injury while you "get fit."

Why Do You Need Different Exercises?

Exercising one body part or system does little to get other parts or systems fit. Doing a good session of stretching every day does a lot for your flexibility, but will not get your cardiovascular system fit. Weight lifting is important for muscle and bone strength, but will not train your sense of balance, which reduces your risk of falls. Getting a good run every day conditions your legs and heart in ways that don't transfer to swimming. That's why good runners often exhaust themselves during long swims, and swimmers during runs, even though both may be aerobically fit.

Each body part, system, and ability gets fit from different kinds of exercise. The principle is called *specificity,* and explains why you need many different activities to be completely fit.

Fit for a Sport vs. Sport for Fitness?

What if you just do one sport and are not interested in other sports? Or any sports? Some people play a sport or do an exercise class just to "get fit," rather than do specific exercises to get in better shape for their sport. For these people, the principle of specificity is still important.

What specificity means to you is that if you do only one kind of activity, such as a regular racquetball game or aerobics class, although it is great exercise, you probably will not be getting fit overall. It's like practicing the tuba. It will not make you a good violin player, even though both are musical skills. You need other exercise for overall health and fitness, even if you regularly "work out" doing one or two activities.

Exercises That "Work" Are Not Always Good for You

Many common exercises will give you the cosmetic results claimed for them. That is, they will shape your muscles, or burn fat. But they may injure your joints and soft tissue. Other exercises work the muscles they claim to work, but not at all in the manner you need in daily life. So they don't do much good, but take up valuable exercise time. You don't need to choose between an exercise that "works" and one that is safe and effective. Plenty of exercises, described below, both "work" and work properly and safely.

Some exercises will make you look better, but are injurious. Other exercises will give you the look you want but without risk of injury.

Aerobic Exercises
Do You Need Step Aerobics?

Cardiovascular workouts of any type improve health and the ability to do physical work. Stepping can be a good cardiovascular exercise with potential to improve strength and muscular endurance of the legs. It also has potential for several injuries.

Stepping down to the rear of the bench, particularly if not done lightly or close enough to the bench, forcibly pulls the Achilles tendon, and can produce painful and slow-healing tendon trauma. Banging down from the bench hard and repeatedly can hurt your calf muscle. Knee injury is also common. How can that be, when physical therapists use stepping for knee rehabilitation? Stepping can help with rehabilitation of one type of knee injury involving the meniscus (the shock-absorbing cartilage "washers" between your upper and lower leg bones). Yet stepping can be injurious on another knee problem—a poorly tracking kneecap that grinds with each step.

Normally, your four quadriceps muscles all pull equally on your kneecap when you move your knee. That makes your knee cap slide up and down in a narrow track in the front of your knee. Stepping can preferentially develop the outer quadriceps muscles more than those on the inside. When the stronger ones on the outside pull more than the weaker ones on the inside, it makes the kneecap track poorly and rub and grind in its groove, causing pain.

Two more problems arise when using a step that is too high. The high degree of knee bending with stepping brings your kneecap in contact with your upper leg bone, even in knees without tracking problems. This can grind your kneecap against your upper leg bone with every step. Many rehabilitation exercises that use a step use a lateral step-up, so that you step to the side rather than the front, avoiding the compression on the kneecap. High benches also magnify impact when stepping down.

How do you know if you will wind up with knee pain or other injuries? One approach is to take a step class and see if it screws up your knees in a few years. Another is to modify how you step. Keep your bench low to reduce knee angle. Step up and down lightly and close to the bench. Incorporate more side step-up moves to reduce the pounding and kneecap compression that forward stepping can produce. An interesting innovation to promote more lateral stepping is to turn the bench so that it faces the front the long way. That way your body can face the instructor while you do lateral stepping. Avoid continuous "repeaters" where you touch down behind the bench repeatedly with the same leg. They are tough on your calf muscles and Achilles tendons.

Problems with Bench Stepping

1. Repeated banging down to the rear of the bench can injure your Achilles tendon and calf muscle.
2. Some people are susceptible to kneecap pain when the kneecap does not slide evenly in its groove, but rubs and grinds. Stepping magnifies this tendency.
3. A high degree of knee bending rubs the kneecap against the upper leg bone with each step, even in knees without tracking problems.

The bottom line on step aerobics: It can help and harm. Modify your stepping to reduce injury potential. Have your knees orthopedically assessed if you get knee pain.

Bench Stepping Modifications

- Step down lightly and close to the bench.
- Avoid banging down with "repeater" steps.
- Incorporate more lateral step-up, stepping to the side rather than the front, to lessen compression on the kneecap.

- Keep your thigh muscles (quadriceps) strong to support your knee, and improve your body's natural shock absorption.
- Keep the step low.

Do You Need Arm Swinging?

Many exercise classes emphasize swinging arms repeatedly overhead and to the side. Although swinging is fun, it burns only a few extra calories and can sometimes cause injury.

The common aerobics class motion of endlessly bending and straightening the elbow with no weights is useless for fitness. If done too much, it may produce a repetitive motion injury. To increase arm strength, you need something that weighs more than your arm, using fewer repetitions.

Swinging the arms behind your body is tough on the front of your shoulder capsule, which is not supposed to be stretched that way. It can cause your shoulder to get out of line, and wear and tear.

The common move of raising the arms repeatedly to the side with the thumbs down, brings a bony prominence at the top of your upper arm bone (the humeral tubercle) crashing into the bony ledge of your shoulder bone above it. That repeatedly squashes structures between them. Ouch. Simply keeping your thumbs turned upward rotates that bony bump of your humeral tubercle out of the way so that it does not impinge against your shoulder bone above it.

Problems with Arm Swinging

1. Repetitive motion injury from endless, uncontrolled bending and straightening.
2. Flailing arms behind the midline of the body can weaken and destabilize the front of the shoulder.
3. Impingement in the shoulder joint often occurs when raising the arm overhead with thumbs turned down.

The bottom line on arm swinging during aerobics: You will make more fitness gains for your arms in the weight room by lifting heavier weights than with repeated swinging. If you enjoy swinging your arms, keep your thumbs facing up, rather than facing down, particularly when you raise your elbows in the "farmer" move. Limit motion backward to no further than the midline of your body. Don't allow momentum to overstretch your shoulders. Lift with control.

Modifications for Arm Swinging

- Keep your thumbs facing up.
- Limit motion backward to no further than the midline of your body.
- Lift your arms with control, rather than speed.

Do You Need Swimming?

Swimming is great for your cardiovascular and muscular systems, and is a low-impact, calorie-burning exercise. Swimming does not use all your muscles (contrary to popular belief) but it is still an excellent exercise for both upper and lower body. The worse you swim, the more calories you burn, and the more your muscles have to work to do the poor, inefficient stroke. Still, taking a stroke mechanics clinic to improve your swimming stroke can increase your enjoyment, the number of laps you can swim, and teach you to swim more safely and comfortably. It is another myth that swimming does not burn fat. If you only swish around, you won't get enough exercise to burn fat. Done as a vigorous exercise, swimming is a fat burner.

Problems with Swimming

1. Swimming is such a good, low-impact, relatively injury-free exercise that it is hard to list problems. If you want to nitpick, you could say that not everyone has a pool handy, and that with poor hygiene, you can get athlete's foot and swimmer's ear.
2. Poor stroke mechanics and bad stretches can lead to shoulder pain.
3. Poor stroke mechanics combined with extreme distance work can result in neck and back pain from twisting movements or over arching vertebral segments.

The bottom line on swimming: Go swimming. Vary your stroke to avoid repetitive-strain injuries. Try arm-only and leg-only work as part of your routine, and swimming with fins for variety and additional leg workouts. Have your stroke checked by a good stroke-mechanics specialist or coach to be able to do more of a workout if you are just a "splasher" or to reduce your chance of mechanical injuries if you pile on the laps.

Modifications for Swimming

- To easily avoid athlete's foot and swimmer's ear, dry your toes and ears well after swimming. Do not remove the protective ear wax that keeps germs out. Ear plugs do not keep much water out of your ears, and there's no need to keep water out. Just dry things afterwards.
- Avoid shoulder-mangling stretches such as lifting arms overhead behind your body.
- Vary your stroke and workout.

"Floor-Work" Exercises

Do You Need Sit-ups?

Sits-ups burn few calories, because you do not do them for long enough for aerobic benefit (even if it *feels* like a long time) and do not remove fat from your abdomen. Done correctly, they strengthen your abdomen, crucial for good posture, back pain control, general activities of daily living, and cosmetic appearance of the midsection. Done incorrectly, they can hurt your back and contribute to poor posture. Chapter 7 has more on abdominal muscles.

Sit-ups, done the traditional way of raising your torso to meet your leg by bending at the hip, work the leg muscles that bend your hip, called hip flexors. The hip flexors lie deep, under your abdominal muscles. You get enough exercise for your hip flexors every day by walking. In most people, the hip flexors are already too strong and tight, causing poor posture and are a common source of back pain (*see* Chapters 20 and 21 on back pain). Sit-ups to develop the hip flexors are useful for sports demanding extreme hip flexor strength— ballet, gymnastics, martial arts, place kicking, but not activities like scuba diving or tennis.

To work your abdominal muscles, do crunches and the often neglected but excellent isometric abdominal exercise explained in the previous chapter on abdominal muscles.

Problems with Sit-ups

1. The traditional sit-up lifts the torso from the floor, bending at the hip. This works muscles that yank on the low back with each repetition, rather than the abdominal muscles.
2. Abdominal muscle exercise, done alone with no back muscle exercise to counter it, can contribute to poor posture and back pain.

The bottom line on sit-ups: Crunches and isometric ab work, not sit-ups, are preferred to improve the abdominal strength and endurance you need to directly benefit your sport, your posture, and part of the support needed by your back.

Modifications for Sit-ups

- Do crunches and other exercises described in Chapter 7 that isolate the abdominal muscles, not sit-ups.
- After doing abdominal muscle exercises, turn over and work your back muscles.

Do You Need Leg Lifts?

Leg lifts to the front, like sit-ups, use more hip flexor muscle action than abdominal muscle work (described above and in Chapter 7). Leg lifts while lying on your side, to work the gluteus medius muscle so popular in exercise classes, do little unless you are debilitated from sedentary living or injury. Your leg is just too light to give the resistance you need for strengthening. Since you can't spot-reduce fat, fat on the side of the hip will not be reduced by any amount of leg lifting.

Side leg lifts while lying down are not a "functional" movement exercise. That means it is not one that you use for your daily life when you move around, or do any sports or recreational activities. Think a minute—when do you use that motion at all? To best work the muscle on the side of your hip, you need to use it during exercise class in the manner that you use it for real. Because of "Specificity of Exercise," the effects on your side hip muscles of doing leg lifts to the side will be different lying down than standing up. Standing leg lifts to the side are more functional.

When you raise your right leg to the side while standing, the gluteus medius on the side of your left hip must work to keep your hip stable. You need strong medius muscles for posture stabilization while walking, running, and any time you need to shift your weight from one leg to the other. That's a lot of reason to develop your gluteus medius in the way it functions.

As far as leg lifts to the back, if there ever was, as Shakespeare supposed, "A deity that shapes our ends," that patron saint of buns is back leg lifts. Lie facedown with your chin on your hands. Lift one leg up slowly with straight knee, hold, then lower. For a tougher exercise, lift both legs together. This action of prone (facedown) hip extension benefits your low back and behind (gluteus maximus muscles), structurally and cosmetically. Don't lift so high that it hurts. If your back hurts no matter how you try it, stop immediately and call for an appointment to be evaluated for back trouble. Another exercise to improve your low back and gluteal muscles is to lie facedown on a chair, bed, couch, bench, or special back apparatus, bending at the waist so that your legs hang off the edge, toward the floor. Then lift your legs until they are in line with your body.

Problems with Leg Lifts

1. Leg lifts to the front use more hip flexor muscle action than abdominal muscle work, and can contribute to poor posture and back pain.
2. Side-lying leg lifts, so popular in exercise classes, do little unless you are debilitated from sedentary living or injury.
3. Side-lying leg lifts are not "functional" movements—you don't use them for any activities. This exercise doesn't benefit your muscles the way you need them.

The bottom line on leg lifts: Leg lifts to the front are not a good abdominal muscle exercise. They use other muscles that pull on the low back. Substitute abdominal crunches instead.

Prone (facedown) hip extension is an excellent back and bun exercise. Strong gluteal muscles are important for shock absorption, and tremendously important for back and knee health.

Side-lying leg lifts are not an effective use of exercise time. They do little to get the hip muscle fit, and what work they do is not in the form that you use in your daily life. Substitute standing leg lifts to the side.

Modifications for Leg Lifts

- Substitute abdominal crunches for leg lifts to the front.
- Do facedown leg lifts for excellent low back and gluteal exercise, important to good posture and back pain control.
- Do leg lifts to the side while standing.

Do You Need Push-ups?

A push-up is a bench press upside down, using your body weight for resistance. You might think that since push-ups use the same three major muscle groups in the same motion as the bench press, it would have the identical training effect. It doesn't because push-ups use your muscles differently. Push-ups also use more muscles.

In the bench press, your hands move freely while your shoulders remain a fixed axis. In the push-up, your hands stay fixed against the floor. Your elbows and shoulders rotate around them. The forces in each joint are different in the two situations. The adaptations are close but separate. Push-ups won't improve your bench press as much as doing bench presses. Specificity again. Also your body weight is often not as much as your bench press weight. You would need to increase your body weight, or add weights to your back by putting weights on your back or having a friend actively resist your push-ups.

Push-ups have many surprising benefits. Although your principle movers are three arm and chest muscle groups, you need a lot of back and abdominal stabilization—the same stabilization so critical for good posture and back pain control. Even if you don't do complete push-ups, just holding the push-up position is very good to get your torso muscles fit for daily life. The push-up uses so many muscles that, if you are pressed for time and have to choose just a few exercises to work as much of your body as possible, do push-ups.

Push-ups work more than your arms. They work your torso-
stabilizing muscles that are important for posture and
back pain control.

If you can't do regular push-ups, there are several, easy, modified push-ups you can start with to build up to regular push-ups. Start by standing up, leaning against a wall, and pushing away. Then work up to a lower starting position, such as the arm of a couch. Then to the floor, resting on your knees. Then regular push-up. When these become easy, and they will with regular work, prop your feet up on a box, then on the couch arm, then finally you may even work up to standing on your hands, against the same wall you started with, to do your advanced incline push-ups.

The bottom line on push-ups: Push-ups are an excellent exercise and have several health and posture benefits. They improve the appearance of your chest and the front of your shoulder and back of your arm. They are a very good exercise to maintain your ability to get up off the floor, more important with every passing year.

Weight Lifting

Weight lifting is good for you. Some people reject lifting for fear of hurting themselves or becoming bulky. Done properly, you reduce your chance of later injury from other activities, and look trimmer. Weight lifting increases your ability to do the physical work of recreational sports and daily activities, like carrying groceries, strengthens and firms you, and increases muscle that burns calories and keeps you warm. Weight lifting increases bone density, which is important for bone health. Weight lifting is one important part of everyone's fitness plan.

Aerobic exercise alone will not increase your lean tissue.
For well-rounded fitness, you need resistance exercises.

Do You Need the Bench Press?

The bench press is a popular lift. In the bench press you lie on your back on a bench, push a weight up from your chest until your arms are straight, then down again to your chest. The bench press works several muscles including those that keep you from falling off the bench. The three muscle groups getting most of the work are the triceps which straighten your arm (located in back of your arm), the round chest muscles called pectoralis major, and the muscles in front of your shoulder called the anterior deltoid.

The bench press can improve size, strength, and endurance of these three muscle groups, but remember specificity. You are pressing up a weight while lying on your back. How often do you need that? In wrestling, in hand-to-hand combat, or anytime something heavy is on top of you and you want to get it off.

The main hazard in bench pressing (aside from dropping the weight on your neck) is lowering the weight so far so that it touches your chest. Many people believe that unless the weight touches the chest, it is not a real exercise. But in most people, the elbows extend too far behind them, stretching the shoulder past a safe range. Such over-stretching can lead to strain, to chronic shoulder problems, and occasionally, shoulder dislocation. Only the barrel-chested, short-armed, power lifters can keep the elbows in line with the body when the weight touches the (large) chest. For the rest of the population, to test how far you should lower the weight, lie on the floor. When your elbows reach the floor, your arms are in line with your shoulder. You may be surprised that the weight is many inches above your chest. But your shoulder joints will not be slowly pried apart.

Problems with Bench Pressing

1. Risk of dropping the weight on your neck.
2. Avoid shoulder trouble by not bringing the weight all the way to your chest. Bring your elbows even with your body, no lower.
3. Tight hips can allow your back to arch when lying on your back.

The bottom line on the bench press: It benefits your physical condition through the usual benefits of weight lifting. It helps you look and feel good. For maximum shoulder safety, limit the range by stopping the weight before your chest. Keep your elbows even with your body; don't let them drop lower. Keep your knees bent for back safety, and stability while lifting.

Modifications for Bench Pressing

- Lift with a spotter.
- Avoid shoulder trouble by not bringing the weight all the way to your chest. Bring your elbows even with your body, no lower.
- Keep your knees bent for back safety, and stability while lifting.

Do You Need the Military Press?

In the military press, or shoulder press, you lift a weight overhead. That is an excellent choice for people who need to hand up heavy boxes overhead, smash a volleyball, or open windows. There is potential for shoulder and back injury if done incorrectly, an even more pressing reason to learn how to do it well. Lifting items overhead is a practical daily life activity. You don't want to hurt yourself putting things up on shelves, or opening windows. People with existing shoulder or back injury need to check with their orthopedists before doing this exercise. Lifting a weight overhead compresses the spine, can worsen a disc problem, and can be tough on rotator cuff injury in the shoulder. If lifting with a barbell, the bar prevents a natural rotation of the arms. Dumbbells work better, allowing natural hand placement. Lift with control, and avoid arching your back when doing this lift. Keep the natural inward curve of the lower back, without exaggerating it.

Sitting is very tough on your back, and sitting while lifting a weight is very, *very* tough on your back. It can be much safer to lift while standing, but even more important to have good posture, because you do not have the aid of the bench to stabilize you. Even more interesting is the connection between tight hip joints and injury from overhead lifting and reaching. When the front of the hip joint is tight, as it often is in most people whether they can feel it or not, the torso can't straighten and arch back in a normal fashion when reaching overhead. The shoulder must overrotate and overcompensate, resulting in rotator cuff injury that is difficult to treat. When the hip is the reason behind the injury, and that is not known or fixed, the shoulder injury keeps coming back. The hipbone really is connected to the shoulder bone.

Problems with the Military Press

1. Lifting a weight overhead compresses the spine, can worsen a disc problem, and can be tough on the shoulder.
2. Lifting with a barbell prevents natural rotation of the arms.
3. Sitting while lifting a weight is very tough on your back.

The bottom line on the military or chest press: It is a good exercise, with direct benefit to activities of daily life. Check with your doctor if you have back or shoulder trouble, before trying the military press. Check your hip and shoulder flexibility to make sure you can lift overhead without overstressing the shoulder. Learn good form, and keep your entire body fit and flexible.

Modifications for the Military Press

- Use dumbbells for more natural hand placement and arm rotation.
- Lift with control.
- Avoid arching your back. Keep the natural inward curve of the lower back, without exaggerating it.

Do You Need Squats?

The squat is an exercise done from a standing position, by bending your knees to a position that looks like sitting in a chair, but without the chair. It is often done holding a weight across the chest or shoulders. Safety of the squat stirs passionate debate. Some insist it is excellent for your body and knees. Others state categorically the squat damages knees. The explanation is simple. The squat has benefits and potential for harm depending how it's done. You can easily modify for the advantages without harming your knees.

Some say the squat is good for you; others say it's bad for you. What's right? Simple.
Done properly, it's very good for you. Done incorrectly, it can injure you.

The squat has many benefits:

- The squat is a multisegment full-body activity, meaning it works many body parts simultaneously. The benefit over isolating each muscle group comes from specificity. From standing, to lifting bags, to getting out of bed, to climbing stairs, to most everything you do, your daily activities are multisegment.
- Squats are good for posture muscles and overall body stabilization.
- Squats raise your capacity for lifting things and accomplishing chores properly. Your back is not made for lifting. The squat trains your legs to do the work. Overall, the squat can be an excellent exercise.
- The squat uses so many muscles that it is a big "bang-for-the-buck" exercise.

The main modification to safeguard knees is to not squat down fully, but stop at a quarter or half way so that your thighs go no farther than parallel to the floor. One way to ensure this is to put a chair behind you, so that your behind will contact the chair at the end of the squat, preventing further lowering. Full squats put high pressure on your knee cartilage. Rising from a full squat twists the leg bones against the cartilage while exerting pressure. Knee problems are occupational injuries of baseball catchers. Once injured, the nonvascular cartilage will not heal. The inflammation may subside, but other times the tear acts as a chronic irritant, inflaming the area until you have surgery. This can be avoided with proper knee posture during squats.

The squat has several variations. One uses no weight at all, except for your own body weight. For many people this is all they need to get a lot of benefit from a simple exercise. Some people, while traveling, do squats in their hotel room, either with their body weight alone, or holding suitcases or wearing a backpack, for a quick, easy workout on the run.

Many people hold a barbell across the back of their neck and shoulders while squatting. Alternatives that are safer for both neck and shoulder include holding weights in each hand, holding the bar across your chest in front of you, or using a machine that places the weight on your shoulders like a horseshoe.

Another way to get most of the benefits of the squat with the least work and risk is to use a "leg sled." You could argue that the leg sled is not a squat at all, but a leg press machine while lying down. There are two main kinds of leg sleds. In one, you lie on your back and push the weight directly upwards with the bottoms of your feet. In the other, you semirecline, pushing the weight diagonally away and upwards. Both of these leg sleds use the same lower body musculature as the squat, and lack the upper body stabilization of the squat. The leg sled done lying down, pushing the weight directly up, keeps most of the compressive forces of the squat off your back, making it a great choice during back pain rehabilitation, and in general.

However you do squats, when returning to the upright position, don't "lock" your knees straight. Maintain the natural inward curve of your lower back. Find a qualified instructor to learn proper form before trying the squat, and start with a broomstick, or light weights until you are well practiced in good form.

Problems with the Squat

1. Full squats put high pressure on your knee cartilage.
2. Rising from a full squat twists and pressures the knee cartilage.
3. Supporting the weight compresses your spine.

The bottom line on the squat: Squats can be excellent for general health and improve your ability in activities of your daily life and recreation, if done correctly. Lift with supervision, keep weights off your neck by holding the bar in front on your chest, or across your shoulders. Keep your back upright, not tilted far forward, and stay above a 90° knee bend.

Modifications for the Squat

- Use a spotter.
- Hold the bar in front on your chest, or across your shoulders, rather than pressing right on the back of your neck.
- Keep your back upright, not tilted forward.
- Keep the natural inward curve of your lower back, without exaggerating it.
- Maintain less than a 90° knee bend.
- Keep your stance wide to reduce stress on your knees.
- Use a leg sled.

Do You Need Leg Machine Exercises?

There are usually two main leg machines. The two seem similar, yet can make a difference in knee health. This topic is one that has seen a lot of debate, and there is still much to learn about how much these two different leg exercises make to your knees. Both work your thigh by straightening the knee against resistance. In one, called the leg press, you push the weight away with the bottom of your feet. In the other, usually called leg extension, you sit with the weight at your ankle, moving your lower leg up and down in an arc. Like the bench press and push-up, these two use the same muscles but with opposite joint dynamics. The second is thought to be tougher on your knees upon full straightening. The first is generally accepted as excellent for your legs without burden to your knee joint. The first one is also more similar to the motions your legs need to do in sports, except for kicking a ball, and used in all daily life movement like walking, running, climbing up and down steps, and getting up out of a chair or bed.

When using the leg press machine, don't bend your knee too much, or lock it straight. An excellent variation of the first leg extension exercise is the leg sled, where you lie on your back and push the weight with the bottoms of your feet. This exercise works your lower body well, without such stress to your back.

Problems with Leg Machines

1. Done improperly, can be tough on the knees.

The bottom line on leg machines: Look for machines where you push the weight with the bottom of your feet, over those where you sit with the weight at your ankle.

Modifications for Leg Machines

- Use machines where you push the weight away with the bottom of your feet (rather than those where you swing the weight up with your ankle).
- Don't "lock" your knees straight.
- Don't bend your knees all the way.

Do You Need Wrist and Ankle Weights?

Swimmers, boxers, and martial artists may use hand, wrist, or ankle weights to add to their workouts. There are two main problems with use of these weights.

Wrist weights for swimmers can contribute to shoulder injury. For punching workouts, the main problem with hand, wrist, and ankle weights is that the resistance is in the wrong direction, which builds the wrong skills.

When swimming, you want to increase your ability to pull backward in an S-shape curve. When punching, you want the power of your punch to go forward. Hand weights for boxing or swimming weigh your arms downward. That preferentially builds muscles and neural pathways that raise your arm upward to resist the downward pull, which is not what you want.

Ankle weights while swimming have similar problems. They throw off your streamline, meaning they throw off your body positioning so that you are no longer horizontal, which reduces your efficiency. Incorrect swimming posture, in turn, makes poor swimming habits by building the wrong neuromuscular patterns. Using weights doesn't really help you swim without them. Tying weights on is also not the safest thing to do in the water, particularly when not wearing a scuba tank.

To improve your swimming or punching ability, you need to increase resistance against your forward progress, not weigh your arms or legs down so that you build patterns that lift upward.

The bottom line on wrist and ankle weights: Don't use them for swimming or punching. They teach you poor form. To improve your swimming, use resistance like tethers, drag suits, and other devices designed to resist your forward progress. For punching skills, use pulleys, or bands that pull your arm directly opposite from the direction you want to develop your punch. If you are punching forward, use a band that holds your arm to the back. If punching diagonally upward, move the band so that it pulls your arm diagonally downward.

Do You Need Balance Exercises?

Who thinks about balance exercises, or even much about balance at all? Yet your ability to balance while walking over uneven terrain or ice can make a big difference to your health and ability to live an active, independent life.

After a three year study of more than 300 senior citizens, researchers at the University of New Mexico in Albuquerque concluded that people were at twice the risk of suffering an injurious fall if they could not balance on one leg for at least 5 seconds.

Many exercises can improve your balance. If you try them, make sure to do them carefully, in a controlled manner, away from nearby objects, and preferably with supervision. If you have past or present ankle, foot, leg, or other problems that affect your balance, see your physician for a supervised balance program first:

- Walk over uneven ground.
- Stand on one foot for increasing periods of time.
- Hop on one foot for increasing periods of time.
- Walk on a line, then walk the line backwards.
- Hop on the line, then hop the line backwards.
- Slalom hop the line, then slalom hop the line backwards.
- Hold a long stretchy band, such as a bungee cord (without the hook). Have a friend hold the other end and pull on it as you walk, then hop the line, to challenge your balance.
- Practice getting up from the floor and back down in a smooth manner. Then repeat without hands. Then repeat holding a package, then with the friend pulling the stretchy band.
- Go ice skating, roller skating, and dancing. Tey Tai-Chi.

More exercises that help balance and control are in the next chapter, "Good and Bad Exercises," in the section on good foot exercises.

The Bottom Line on 10 Popular Exercises (and one that you may not have thought about)

Step Aerobics. Can help and harm. Modify stepping to reduce injury potential. The general fitness from this activity benefits your general health directly, and ability in your chosen sports indirectly.

Arm Swinging During Aerobics. Has potential for repetitive strain injury, and gives little extra exercise. If you enjoy swinging your arms, keep your thumbs facing up when lifting upward. Limit motion backward to no further than the midline of your body. Lift with control. Don't confuse momentum with strength. To tone or strengthen your arms, you will make more gains through weight training.

Swimming. Good, low-impact aerobic exercise that works both upper and lower body muscles. Vary your workout and have more fun with fins, kickboards, paddles, and other toys.

Sit-ups. Substitute crunches and isometric ab exercises for sit-ups, to improve the abdominal strength and endurance that directly benefits your posture, your ability to go long days without back pain, and for sports and recreation. Don't do only ab exercises without turning over and doing back exercises. Abs are only part of the support you need. Alone, they can just make you slouch more.

Leg Lifts. Leg lifts lying facedown are a great back and bun exercise. For front and side lifts, it is better to do them standing than lying down. Using a band or weight on your legs will improve your leg strength, endurance, and firmness more than using body weight alone.

Push-ups. Uses many upper-body and torso stabilization muscles. Great for strength and posture. More "bang for the buck" than many other exercises.

Bench Press. For shoulder safety, limit the range by stopping the weight before your elbows go too far behind you.

Military Press. Learn proper form for safety. Check with your doctor if you have back or shoulder trouble.

The Squat. Squats can be excellent for general health, shaping the lower body, and many sports. Lift with supervision, keep weights off your neck, keep your back upright, not tilted forward, and stay above a 90° knee bend.

Leg Machines. Look for machines where you push the weight with the bottom of your feet, over those that have you sit with the weight at your ankle.

Balance Exercises. Balance exercises are important to preventing falls, and improving your overall fitness for an active, independent life. Make sure to practice with supervision, and when there is no danger of falling onto nearby objects.

Getting Fit Has Many Components

Fitness has many different components. To improve your fitness and health, you need many different activities that work all your different systems and body parts. Weight lifters may not be lowering their risk of heart trouble if they never work their cardiovascular system too. People who just play tennis need to add weight lifting, stretching, and something with a longer-duration aerobic component. You may be in good shape, yet at risk of falls from poor stability and poor balance.

Getting in shape for any specific sport or activity requires doing that particular activity, and exercising the muscles used in the specific skills. Runners may be in great shape for running, but may easily poop out when trying to swim.

Doing many different exercises doesn't mean drudgery; it can be fun. Doing different things helps liven up old routines and prevent burnout. For now you're off to a good start to fitness. Make an appointment with yourself, determine a variety of exercises you enjoy for each different system and body part, get out there, and enjoy getting fit.

9

Good and Bad Exercises

He shall not alter it, nor change it, a good for a bad, or a bad for a good.

—Leviticus 27:10

Some exercises are good for you. Many popular moves will make you look good, but will eventually injure your joints. Others do nothing at all. How can you know what is good and what is hype? This chapter looks at a few of each, from top to toe.

Your Neck

Your neck has a lot to do all day. It moves constantly and supports the weight of your head. The strength, flexibility, and posture of your neck can make a big difference to your comfort and energy levels.

Poor neck posture from tight, weak neck muscles often brings on pain between your shoulders, under the shoulder blades, around your neck, and down the tops of your shoulders. The most common poor neck posture is standing and sitting with your chin and head forward.

Problematic Neck Exercises

The vertebrae of your neck are not shaped for motion through a circular path. Neck rolls (head rolls) are tough on your neck over time.

Two classic exercises press your neck into extreme forward positions—the overhead bicycle where you churn your legs in the air with all your weight on your shoulders and neck, and the plow, where you lie with your legs in the air over your head and all your weight on your shoulders and neck. Both of these force the neck too far forward, putting pressure on the discs, and overstretching the long ligament down the back of your neck. When ligaments stretch out, they don't return to their healthy length, weakening the neck. A permanent forward head may result, giving you funny posture and upper back pain.

You're better off without doing the "plow" stretch. There are better ways to simultaneously have a stroke and herniate discs in your neck.

Other exercises that make a forward head posture worse include pulling your neck forward for abdominal work, craning and tensing your neck while lifting weights, and tipping your neck forward while lifting or pulling a bar in back of your neck. The traditional "lat pull-down" where you pull a bar down in back of your neck forces your neck into bad posture, and does not even work your "lats," the large latissimus dorsi muscles of your back and sides, in the line of the muscle fibers. Modifying this exercise by pulling the weight in front of your neck, rather than behind it, changes it into a good exercise.

Healthy Neck Exercises

Strengtheners. To strengthen the muscles of your upper back that contribute to good head posture, lie facedown, arms out at your sides, and gently, slowly, lift your arms and upper body from the floor, and hold. Then slowly lower and repeat. Work up to 10 repetitions at a time. Don't do anything that hurts.

When lifting or pulling weights, keep the weight in the front of your neck, not behind it.

Stretches. For a healthy neck range of motion, don't roll your head around. Just look down, look up, look left, look right, and tip each ear to each shoulder. Keep your shoulders down, not up in your ears.

Figure 9.1. Some exercises force your neck into a forward posture, straining your neck. A forward head posture can eventually become a habit. A slouching forward head posture is not good for you, so why practice it in a gym?

Posture Exercises. To correct poor head posture, practice pulling your chin in and head back until your ears center over your shoulders. Keep your gaze looking forward, not up or down, just pull back. Try it for 10 counts to start, then learn to hold the good posture all day.

For more good neck strengtheners, stretches, and posture exercises, *see* Chapter 21.

Your Arms, Shoulders, and Chest

Strong upper bodies look sexy and can carry more things, more easily, with less chance of injury.

Problematic Arm, Shoulder, and Chest Exercises

Swinging the arms in aerobics class was mentioned in the previous chapter. Two shoulder injuries appear most often. The first from swinging your arms too hard and far from front to back. The front of the shoulder capsule, constitutionally too weak to withstand such trauma, forcibly stretches past a safe range. In the second, called "The Farmer," you turn your thumbs down, and lift both elbows. This action brings a structure on your upper arm bone, technically called the humeral tubercle, directly under the bony ledge of your shoulder bone, technically called the acromion, squashing the cushiony sac between them called a bursa. Over time this can produce what is technically called "An Injury," known as bursitis.

When doing the bench press, many people are taught to touch the bar to their chest, but with so many different arm lengths and chest widths, that is not for everyone. For most people, it allows the elbows to lower too far down, harmful to the front of the shoulder.

Swimming is great for your upper body in general but doesn't work all your muscles. Swimming preferentially ignores your biceps and the muscles called external rotators, that turn your arm in a thumb-upward position like a hitchhiker, while building internal rotators that rotate the arm thumb-downward. The underpowered external rotators may destabilize the shoulder, at times contributing more to swimmer's shoulder than the repetitive action of swimming itself.

Certain stretches can be injurious to your shoulders. Many exercisers seem to reproduce wartime torture techniques. They clasp their hands together behind them, and yank their arms up overhead in back. Swimmers routinely do this for a greater range of motion, which can improve swimming speed. The price can be shoulder instability and susceptibility to long-term injury. Ironically, when pain develops, they are often told, "Gee, a shoulder injury and you're a swimmer. It must be the repetitive strain of swimming, so you had better stop the swimming for a while." Meanwhile, it was not necessarily the swimming, but the stretching. The poorly advised person continues to stretch, and no longer has the muscle-building activity of swimming. Strong shoulder muscles help to counteract the laxity and instability that poor stretching technique can produce. The unstable shoulder joint continues to rub, clank, and hurt.

Sometimes, it's not the shoulder exercise (like swimming) that wrecks the shoulder, but the damaging shoulder stretches done.

Another popular, but problematic shoulder stretch is forcibly holding your arm in back of your body by pressing the side of your arm against a wall. This overstresses the front of the shoulder capsule, and overstretches parts that are not healthy to stretch. It also does not stretch the front of your chest, a stretch that a majority of people need.

Many people sit round-shouldered, which shortens the muscles, creating a vicious cycle of shortening and round-shouldered posture. This posture can create back and neck pain. The shortening can continue until the person's arms turn inward, so that their thumbs face the body, instead of hanging forward, naturally.

Good Arm, Shoulder, and Chest Exercises

Strengtheners. The rotator cuff muscles of the shoulder are usually neglected. People work their deltoids and chest and back, but it is your four rotator cuff muscles that stabilize your arm and shoulder. Working the surrounding muscles but not the rotator cuff can allow the top of your upper arm bone to push and grind against your shoulder capsule. One good exercise for the rotator cuff is to lie on your left side, with your right elbow bent and a hand weight held near your navel. Hold a small hand weight in your right hand. Keep your elbow close to your body, but not touching it. You can use a towel as a spacer and elbow rest. Lift the weight up toward the ceiling, then lower. Then, while still lying on your left side, switch the weight to the left hand and lift. Switch sides after each set.

For a good rotator cuff exercise while standing, get a length of rubber tubing, and secure it at elbow height from anything that will hold it while you pull. Turn sideways, elbow bent. Use a towel between your elbow and waist as a spacer and elbow rest. Pull the tubing, making sure that you do not pull so hard, or so far, that it hurts. Turn facing the other way and pull in the other direction. Work up to about 10 repetitions on each side.

The best strengtheners for the upper body use weights, whether dumbbells, weight machines, or your body weight. Waving your arms in an aerobics class won't do it. Your arm does not weigh enough by itself to provide the resistance your muscles need to get stronger. Try the various machines, or lift dumbbells, packages, yourself, or willing friends, to exercise your biceps, triceps, and shoulder. The upper back exercises, described in Chapters 20 and 21 on back and neck pain, are also good for shoulder stabilization.

When doing the bench press, keep your elbows in line with your shoulders, not lower. A good way to check this is to lie on the floor and lower your elbows until they touch the floor. That is where to stop your bench press, even if the bar does not touch your chest. Read more on the bench press, push up, and military press in the previous chapter.

Figure 9.2. When exercising your arms and shoulders, remember your rotator cuff muscles. Good rotator cuff muscles are important to the health of your shoulder joint and for normal arm functioning.

Stretches. To stretch your arms, shoulders, and chest, move through a gentle range of motion in all directions. Don't yank your arms up behind you overhead.

Combination Stretch/Posture Exercise. To stretch the front of the chest and shoulder, stand in a doorway and hold your arm out to your side, bending your elbow 90° so that your fingers face the ceiling, hand forward, as if calling someone to a stop. Press the inside of your elbow against the doorway, then gently turn your body away from your arm. You should feel a pleasant stretch in the front of your chest, just below the shoulder. This stretch also brings the shoulder back in line with the body, demonstrating proper shoulder posture. Most people stand round-shouldered, with their shoulders forward of the midline of their body.

Your Abdomen

Abdominal muscles run down the front of you from your ribs to your pelvic bones. One of their duties is to hold some tension all the time to keep you from arching too far backward during normal standing and sitting. Muscles running along your back work similarly to

Figure 9.3. For a good chest and shoulder stretch, press the inside of your bent elbow against a doorway or wall, then gently turn away from that arm. This is good for improving posture. Do this instead of yanking your arms up behind you, which is tough on your shoulder joint.

keep you from slouching over forward. Weakness in your back and/ or ab muscles allow you to sit and stand in ways that slowly injure you without knowing it. Benefits from improved abdominal muscles, and specific exercises were covered in Chapter 7 on abdominal muscles.

Problematic Abdominal Exercises

Leg lifts and full sit-ups don't use your ab muscles as much as they use another set of muscles that bend your hip. Overworking these hip flexors is tough on the back.

Another problem with ab exercises occurs when you strengthen your abs too much until your weaker back muscles can't counter the pull from the front. Abs create an important support structure for your torso, but they are not the entire support. When you exercise your abs, also work your back muscles with the exercises described in the earlier paragraphs on backs, and Chapters 20 and 21 on back pain. Without adding back exercises to your ab routine, your tight abs can pull you too far forward, resulting in poor posture and back pain. That's why "ab-only" classes, although popular, are not as helpful as you would think. These classes need to incorporate back exercises as well.

Leaning sideways from side to side while holding hand weights is not an ab exercise. It does not benefit your back and does not tone or reduce your midsection. The muscles in play here are called "hip hikers," used in walking to keep the swinging leg from dragging on the ground.

The standing torso twist from side to side is not an ab exercise. Holding a weight on the shoulders and twisting can generate momentum greater than the supporting structures of your back and knee can safely absorb.

Figure 9.4. The torso twist is not an ab exercise and can be hard on your back.

Good Abdominal Exercises

Crunches, not sit-ups, are good exercise for your abs. Even better is a much neglected, but needed isometric ab exercise. All are fully described in Chapter 7 on abdominal muscles.

Your Back

A common medical prescription for back pain—"Gee, you should get more exercise"—is true but vague. Many exercises popular at gyms and exercise studios cause more harm than good, and can directly injure your back over time without you being aware of the harm in progress. *See* Chapter 20 for more on why your back can hurt and Chapter 21 for what exercises to do.

Problematic Back Exercises

A few bad exercises now and then usually do little damage, but give it a chance. Like smoking, the repeated, forced nature of the exposure can harm at a rate faster than your body can repair.

Some tough-on-your-back exercises are weight lifting while leaning over unsupported from the waist, straight-leg dead lifting, forced repetitive back arching like "donkey kicks" that swing the leg overhead from a hands and knees position, and forced repetitive back bending like toe touches from a stand or swinging elbows down to opposite knees.

Leaning over at the waist for toe touches stretches your back and hamstrings, but it is not a good stretch for regular use. Although it feels great when back muscles are tight, it is tough on your back in the long run.

A bad exercise, like straight-leg dead lifting, may not hurt
when you're doing it, but can still injure you over years.
Just give it a chance.

Good Back Exercises

You can do many things in your daily routine to make your back more injury resistant. Strength, posture, and stretching for the back are so important that there are two chapters devoted to explaining everything in detail. *See* Chapters 20 and 21.

Important points to remember when exercising your back are to keep the natural inward curve of your lower back. Don't let it reverse into the shape of the letter C when sitting or lifting. For example, when rowing with pulleys or a rowing machine, don't sit and pull with a rounded back.

When using free weights, don't lean over unsupported. When lifting dumbbells, support your body weight by resting one hand on your knee, and lifting with the other hand, or by leaning against an incline bench.

Good range of motion in all the directions your back bends helps prevent back pain. Stretch through your back's range of motion slowly as part of your regular routine. A safer way to stretch your back than standing or sitting toe touches is to lie on your back and bring one bent leg to your chest at a time.

Figure 9.5. Some common exercises can be hard on your back even if you are in good shape. You know that bending over to lift is bad for your back, even more so with straight legs. It does not magically become good for you in a gym, even as a stretch. It can cumulatively stress and damage your back. Straight-leg deadlifting, although popular, has more risks than benefits.

Your Legs

Strong legs are important for your daily life activities. It's important to exercise your legs until they are strong enough to lift things, instead of using your back. Your back was not made for lifting. Doing regular leg exercise dramatically reduces the effects of aging. You may have seen aged people too weak to rise from a chair unaided. This is not usually an inescapable feature of aging; it is usually an avoidable problem of deconditioning. These people benefit greatly from weight training programs, and are able to make dramatic improvements to their mobility and independent living.

Your legs have posture. This posture is not just something you are born with. You can change your leg posture so that it is good or bad. Bad leg posture can increase wear and tear on your knees and hips.

Problematic Leg Exercises

The hurdler's stretch twists your knee sideways with possibility of knee ligament damage. The double hurdler's stretch is worse. In that still-common stretch, you sit on the floor on your heels, both knees bent, sometimes with both feet facing outward, and lean far backward. This is hard on the back, and worse on the knees. Full squats (sitting on your heels) and duck walks are tough on the knees. They pry the

Figure 9.6. When doing back or shoulder exercises, don't bend over unsupported. Always support your upper body weight. It's not wimpy, and it's not just for people with back problems. It's for anyone who does not want to have a back problem.

knee joints open, particularly if you have heavy thighs, and can damage knee cartilage.

The hurdler's stretch is not recommended. It twists your knee behind you. Modify by keeping both legs in front of you, one bent at the knee.

Good Leg Exercises

In general, it's easy to exercise your legs.

Strengtheners. Walk, run, ride a bike, ski, carry things, go up and down stairs, swim with fins, get up and walk away from the TV. Try it. It works. These exercises use your body weight as resistance. Adding more weight through safe weight lifting can lead to better gains in leg strength. Weight lifting for your legs can be done with weight machines, or other equipment.

A fun isometric exercise for your legs that uses your body weight for resistance is called the "ski-sit." Put your back against a wall, feet away from the wall. Slide down until you are in a position as if you were sitting in a chair, suspended in space. Make sure your knees are right over your ankles, not past them. Hold. Time how long you can endure.

Figure 9.7. The hurdler's stretch is not good for your knees even if you are flexible. Curling your back forward is also not good for your back. You know that you do not want a round-shouldered, slouching forward posture, so why practice it in a gym?

Stretches. To stretch the back of your legs, lie on your back and straighten one leg up overhead and hold. Or stand with one heel propped up on a chair keeping the inward curve of your lower back, and sticking your behind out a little. Do these instead of the bent-over toe touch, which is tough on your back.

For toe touches, substitute lying down with one leg overhead, or one leg on a chair, rather than the bent-over toe touch.

Figure 9.8. The ski-sit is a fun, isometric exercise for your legs.

Another important, but often forgotten stretch, is for your iliotibial band or "I.T. Band." Your I.T. band extends down the side of your hip to your knee. Tight I.T. bands can lead to knee pain, and even change the way you walk, which leads to other problems. To stretch your I.T., stand sideways at arm's-length from a wall, right hand touching the wall. Cross your left leg in front of your right. Push your hips forward, then toward the wall. Make sure you are not leaning backwards, or you will not feel a stretch. Hold for about 30 seconds, then switch sides.

Posture Exercises. The muscles of your legs can be weak, tight, or even overstretched, allowing your legs to turn and slump from natural and healthy alignment.

1. Stand in front of a full-length mirror. See if your knees slump inside the line between your hips and ankles, or look "knock-kneed." Practice pulling slightly out with your outer leg muscles so that you can hold your knees straight ahead, and aligned over your ankle bones, when you stand and walk.
2. Look in the mirror, standing with both feet straight ahead. See if your kneecaps "look" at each other, or face away from each other. Practice holding your knees straight ahead, and aligned over your ankle bones when you stand and walk.

Figure 9.9. Remember to stretch your iliotibial or "I.T." band, a fibrous band of supporting tissue which extends down the side of your hip to the outside of your knee. Tight I.T. bands can lead to knee pain, even change the way you walk.

Your Feet

Your feet? Who thinks about exercising their feet? Yet your feet help determine if you will get through your day with easy energy, or limp home hurting and tired. Without strong, flexible, well-balanced musculature of your feet and ankles, problems can occur:

- Standing and walking with poor foot and ankle posture changes how you distribute your weight across your ankles, knees, and hips. That creates extra pressures, shock, and wear.
- Weak ankles are prone to recurring sprains.
- Tight, inflexible feet and ankles may be more likely to cramp.
- If your big toe joint does not bend pliably when walking, it throws off your gait, and pushes the posture of your head and trunk forward. Your low back muscles and discs bear the brunt.
- Injured or weak feet and ankles do not have good motor control or proprioception. (Proprioception means knowing where you are in space.) They cannot react to changes in balance and footing quickly enough. You may turn your ankle before your body recognizes and corrects for it. Good foot and ankle exercises can retrain kinesthetics, motor control, and balance awareness.
- Tight Achilles tendons and calf muscles hobble your gait, making you take short steps. They are more likely to strain when you try to walk or run faster.
- The commonest cause of ongoing ankle pain or recurring ankle sprains is incomplete rehabilitation from the last time.
- When the bottoms of your feet get too tight, that contributes to a condition where tissues attached to the heel irritate the heel because they pull on it too tightly with every step. This is called plantar fasciitis. *Plantar* means the bottom of your foot (that you "plant" on the ground) and *fasciitis* is an inflamation of the fascia, the fibrous connective tissue spanning the bottom of your foot. Untreated plantar fasciitis can lead to heel spurs. Your heel gets so irritated with all the pulling that, like an oyster, it grows a "pearl" of a bony spur.
- Your feet have posture. Many cases of "flat feet" and "pigeon toes" are not unchangeable hereditary conditions, just poor foot and ankle posture.

Your feet contribute to your posture and shock absorption,
important to preventing back, neck, knee, and hip pain.

Problematic Foot Exercises

There seem to be very few problematic foot exercises, mostly
because few people bother to exercise their feet and ankles at all.
Bad foot exercises haven't had a chance to become popular. Mostly,
bad shoes (more common than you would think) and lack of good
exercises lead to foot problems. *See* Chapters 20 and 21 on back and
neck pain for more on proper shoes.

One common exercise that weakens the ankle is sitting in a "butter-
fly position" with the soles of your feet touching, but with your knees
high. This stretches the sides of your ankles too far, loosening them.
The loose, destabilized ankle becomes prone to recurring sprains.

Ankle sprains, particularly recurring ankle sprains, usually
come from ankles overstretched on the sides, allowing
too much movement. Weak or injured ankles also do not
have normal "knowledge" and control of balance.
They cannot correct for a sudden trip quickly enough.
Instead of righting you, these weak, slow,
overstretched, and "unaware" ankles let you fall.

Good Foot Exercises

Strengtheners. More successful than high-top shoes, taping,
orthotics, and bracing in preventing ankle sprains, are strong ankle
muscles. Most sprains come from rolling over the outside edge of
your foot, so that the outside edge turns down. That motion is called
inversion. While sitting with no weight on your foot, identify that
motion. That's what you want to avoid in stretching and exercising.
The opposite motion, where you lift the outside edge of your foot
up, is a motion called *eversion.* (Don't confuse eversion with prona-
tion, where you let your arch flatten.) Your everter muscles are main
muscles to strengthen:

1. Loop a short, heavy rubber tube or bungee cord around both feet. Roll the outside edges of your feet outward and upward and hold. Repeat. Gradually increase the number you can do.
2. With the same tube, keep the heels together and point the toes away from each other, resisted by the tube. Hold and repeat.
3. Repeatedly press the side of your ankle upward against a wall and hold for 10 counts. Repeat at different angles.
4. Get a towel and any 5–10-pound weight, even a big book. Set the weight on the towel, and your bare foot next to it. Pivot on your heel to slide the towel with your toes. Do both directions, pivoting inward and outward.

To strengthen the bottoms of your feet, pull a weighted towel toward you by scrunching it with your toes.

Posture Exercises. Some people allow their arches to sag too flat or, occasionally, roll to the side until they are too arched. Others might have weak leg muscles, allowing their stance to toe in or out.

Think of your feet as the front end alignment of your car.
The tires are your feet and can have posture problems
in three directions—"caster, camber, and of course, toe."

---

1. Look in a mirror and see if your feet tilt, making your arches too high or low. Practice pressing and lifting the arch while keeping the rest of the sole on the floor. See how the muscles work on the inside and outside of your leg to do that.
2. Look in the mirror and see if your toes point in or out. Practice walking with your toes straight ahead.

Don't be fooled by just looking at the bottoms of your shoes for wear patterns. It is true that the bottoms of your shoes can tell a lot if they are completely worn on one side. But it is natural to heel-strike slightly to the side first, then roll to an even position. Shoes with slight wear on the outside heel do not necessarily mean that you are not walking "squarely." To determine that, you need to watch yourself in a mirror or, better yet, have a trained gait mechanics specialist give you a full walking evaluation.

Figure 9.10. Good foot exercises can do a lot for your overall health. The strength and posture of your feet and ankles has a big influence on your chance of some kinds of foot, ankle, knee, and hip pain, and your risk of ankle sprains.

Balance/Kinesthetics Exercises. Among the many balance and kinesthetic exercises you can do, here are just a few:

1. Bounce and catch a ball while standing on one leg.
2. Catch a ball thrown against the wall.
3. Balance on one foot. Repeatedly rise to the toe and lower, then bend the knee and rise again. Balance on tiptoe by pressing on the big and second toe, not wobbling on the outsides of your feet.
4. When your strength and balance have progressed, hop on one foot along a line on the floor.
5. Try to slalom the line hopping.

Floppy Foot Exercises. It is important to learn how to not "hold" tension in your feet and ankles. This leads to cramps and rigidity, and reduces shock absorption. The floppy foot exercises are explained in great length in Chapter 30 on leg cramps. To summarize here, they consist of being able to separate your foot from muscular control until you can take your ankle in both hands, and shake the foot so that it flops with each shake.

1. Try it with your hand first, which is easier. Take one wrist in the other hand, and shake it.
2. Now duplicate the floppy, tensionless movement in your feet. It will pay.

Stretches. Flexible feet allow healthy range of motion when walking, and reduce chance of strains and tears.

- An important stretch keeps your toes, particularly your big toe, flexible. Stand with one foot in back of you, and lift that heel as you do in walking, bending the toes. Hold and repeat. Then stretch your toes in the other direction, by pressing the top of your toes against the floor behind you, or your hands.
- You can stretch your Achilles tendon and calf several ways. Carefully standing backwards on a step, let one heel hang off, and press downward. Do this with your leg bent, with it straight, and with the leg straight and your body leaning forward, sticking your behind out. You can also stand facing a wall, one foot in back, toes straight ahead, and lean your hips toward the wall. Do both legs.
- Point and bend your ankle up and down to increase range of motion.
- Stretch the bottoms of your feet by pulling your toes back firmly and holding. This is a good one to do in the morning to help treat and prevent plantar fasciitis, and to get your feet ready for the day.

Work Both Sides for Stabilization

When you work one muscle group, it is important to work the opposite muscles. That way you do not overpower your body in one direction, leaving you vulnerable to poor posture and strains over the long run.

A workout that balances work in each direction is sometimes called a "push-pull" workout. When you push one way in lifting, you also do exercises that pull the other way. It's not necessary to immediately follow each "push" exercise with its corresponding "pull." Simply do them in the same day's workout.

- When you work your arms, work both your biceps and your triceps.
- Match bench presses with rows (pulling the weight toward your chest).
- Balance lateral arm raises with lateral pull downs.
- When you work your legs, do exercises for the quadriceps muscles in front, and your hamstring muscles in back.
- After working your calf muscles, remember exercises for your shins.
- When you do ab curls, also do back extensions (explained in Chapter 21 on back pain).
- If you do wrist curls, do one set toward your palm and another set toward the back of your hand.

Choose Good Exercises

This chapter barely touched on a few of the good, the bad, and the peculiar of the many exercises you may encounter. See your physician before starting your exercise program. Lift weights with supervision. Improve your health and fitness by choosing good exercises and sticking with them. Have fun.

10

Just Overdo It, and What to Do When You Do Too Much

First, don't smoke to excess; second, don't drink to excess;
third, don't marry to excess.

—Mark Twain

Usually the problem is getting people to exercise at all. Occasionally the opposite is true. Excess physical activity once in a while is fun, often productive and exciting. But what if you do too much, too soon, too often? Sore muscles for the weekend warrior, and chronic injury and burnout for the exercise obsessed, are the wages of those who "Just Overdo It."

Just Overdo It

Sedentary people just deciding to get in shape typically begin an exercise program with happy expectation. They expect a year's results in a few frantic weeks. That approach is not without its place. The initial infatuation with exercise gets you started. But rather than softly making exercise a lifetime friend, overenthusiastic new exercisers pound themselves mercilessly. A few weeks later they are "beat up from the feet up," irritable, and sometimes, injured. Their plan is not novel or fun anymore. They've had enough—enough pounding and enough proof that exercise wasn't for them anyway.

Other people exercise regularly. Then one day they decide to better their physical condition by bumping up their routines. To warp speed.

Still others don't exercise. They occasionally lug a heavy cooler in and out of their trunk to go play softball, or go skiing. Monday morning they don't call in sick to work because they're too sore to pick up the phone.

How Much Is Too Much?

How do you know if you're overdoing it? According to basketball coach Dean Smith, "If you make every game a life-and-death proposition, you're going to have problems. For one thing, you'll be dead a lot."

Usually though, the clues are not so obvious. With any overenthusiastic, unaccustomed exercise you can overdo, even with activity seeming mild to a more conditioned exerciser.

Several things turn doing into overdoing. Being out of shape for the activity, insufficient warm-up, and too little rest between exercise sessions are key. Exercisers also sometimes starve themselves, hoping to increase weight loss.

Spoken warnings of impending excess may include the phrase, "I used to be pretty good at this . . ." heard just before activities enjoyed long ago, with no conditioning since then.

The Short-Term Overdo

Soreness

You don't exercise often, but one day you go out and have a great time, go home, wake up the next morning, and get your first clue. You've got delayed onset muscle soreness (DOMS). DOMS isn't usually dangerous and isn't permanent. It just feels that way. It's beyond the scope of this book to detail the theorized mechanisms and consequences of DOMS. In brief, unaccustomed mechanical stress leads to a cascade of events including damage to the proteins in your muscle fibers, and a big inflammatory response. You're stiff, sore, and weak for one to three days. You've just overdone it.

Acute Injury

Sometimes you haven't just overdone it, you've charbroiled it. Beside the sometimes unavoidable Frisbee in the face, acute injury commonly results from being too out-of-shape, or without sufficient flexibility for the intensity and range of motion you needed for the activity. This is the way you strain muscle fibers and twist joints into positions that harm them.

The Long-Term Overdo

Physical and Mental Decline

Up to a point, regular physical exercise enhances health, athletic ability, and feelings of energy. Findings from mental health research indicate positive mood change, increased intellectual function, and improved self-concept, although causal links are not known for sure.

Overdoing exercise reverses the situation. Athletic ability, energy, physical health, and state of mind suffer. "Fatigue," Napoleon observed, "makes cowards of us all."

Diminished physical performance sometimes drives frustrated exercisers to push harder to offset the decline. The overtraining cycle of fatigue, depression, and overdoing continues.

Chronic Injury

Overtraining overloads your musculoskeletal system. In plain English, you wear something out. The resulting injury can cause other injuries later on. Injuries that throw off how you walk and stand eventually stress previously healthy structures into new injuries. Some injuries you might not be aware of. These unrecognized injuries quietly build, decreasing performance and increasing long-range orthopedic consequences. Other, painful injuries, although outwardly more worrisome, can be helpful because they limit further overdoing (except in the pleasure-impaired).

Immune Decline

Studies of immune function seem to show a trend where moderate exercise possibly helps immune function, but intense overtraining can suppress the immune system. Most of the changes so far identified are small, variable, and temporary. It is still not known if these changes increase the risk of recurrent infection or other diseases during periods of extreme ultratraining.

Obsession

The exercise-obsessed person panics at the thought of missing a workout. They are certain that missing their day's pounding means undoing years of hard work. (This phenomenon is not limited to exercise. It includes just about any activity that you overdo.) Although their bodies and physical progress would be better off with rest and recovery time, they go at it every day. Their lack of progress spurs them to further excess. A frustrated cycle perpetuates of obsession, not enough recovery time, overdoing, and lack of progress.

Burn Out

We've all done it. Some have done it plenty of times—start out great guns then fizzle. The burnout syndrome can be summed up by the progression "Triweekly, Try weekly, Try weakly."

How to Just Not Overdo It

Sunday soldiers and chronic exercise abusers are well researched in sport science, in part because they're so common. The literature reports several strategies to avoid overdoing.

Identify Problems

The point where "doing" becomes "overdoing" is difficult to define. What aspect of your activity do you overdo? Have you built up slowly to the task or did you just plunge in? Is your activity too intense for your abilities? Is your intensity level all right but without enough rest? Do you rest and train moderately yet still suffer injuries? In that case, it may not be overuse but improper use. Not making progress? Is it lack of rest or not the right exercises? If you're still tired and miserable given an appropriate and safe program, you may need to change the kind of exercise you do. Try a different activity. This time make it one you like.

Modify

If it hurts when you do it, don't do it. Reduce the mileage, the amount of weight, the frequency, the intensity—whatever makes it too much—and then keep moving, but at a safe and sane level.

Avoid Misuse

Were you too out of shape to carry the cooler or haul up the anchor, or did you just lift wrong and screw up your back? Injury may stem not from overdoing, but misuse, bad gait, poor lifting technique, or problematic exercises. Read about a few of these problems in Chapter 9, "Good and Bad Exercises," and Chapters 20 and 21, "Back and Neck Pain." If misuse is the problem, modify your technique, equipment, or gait. Figure out which injuries you get from overuse and which from misuse.

Train in Cycles

Do you work out too much? The sport science literature is pretty clear that rest is crucial for physical improvement. With rest between sessions, you avoid the problems of overdoing, while increasing your physical ability more than possible by training every day. Alternating days of exercise and rest is called exercise cycling and periodization. Try it.

Top athletes don't work out every day. Athletes successfully training for strength usually lift three or four days each week. They don't practice their major heavy lifts like the press, pulls, or squat more than two days per week. During competitions they then cut back overall training to 1–3 days per week. Top runners allow days of rest between long runs and taper their mileage before races.

Get in Shape

Maybe you don't work out enough to be in shape for the occasional activity you do. Developing some semblance of fitness increases the variety of activities you can do without later paying the piper. Stick with at least a mild exercise program all year, not just in sports season.

Warm Up

Do you fling into activities without warming up? Well, warm up first. Warm-up, just as it sounds, means raising your body temperature. Warm-up is not stretching, arm waving, or rising up and down on tiptoe. Those activities do not raise body temperature. Use large muscle rhythmic activities like walking, slow jogging, swimming, or cycling to warm up. Be warm enough to sweat before you stretch or begin activity. *See* Chapter 5 on warm-ups.

Enjoy Yourself

Do you enjoy the exercise you do? A major point to consider is "Are you happy?" Make your program one that satisfies your soul along with your body. If you hate your program, chances are you won't stick with it however well intentioned.

At the other end of the continuum are those disciplined beings that slog through misery for the results, never mind the painful journey. Try enjoying yourself. Find aspects of exercise that you like. Incorporate rest periods. You'll find your performance improves with a day off in between exercise bouts.

If, on the other hand, you enjoy obsessing, go ahead and obsess. Identify and modify aspects that injure your body, social life, or happiness. Then, if overdoing is really for you, then just overdo it. Remember to reassess periodically. And go see a movie sometimes.

How to Just Not Overdo It

Identify Problems. Have you built up gradually enough? Does your intensity level suit your fitness level? Do you get enough rest? Do you like the exercise you do?

Modify. If it hurts when you do it, don't do it. Reduce the mileage, amount of weight used, frequency, intensity, or whatever parameter makes it too much.

Avoid Misuse. Is it overuse or misuse? Bad gait? Poor lifting technique? Bad exercises?

Train in Cycles. Rather than training every day, rest between sessions. You'll avoid the problems of overdoing, while increasing your fitness.

Get in Shape. Developing some semblance of fitness increases the variety of activities you can do without later paying the piper.

Warm Up. Warm-up, just as it sounds, means raising your body temperature. It is not stretching, arm waving, or rising up and down on tiptoe. Be warm enough to sweat before you stretch or begin exercise.

Enjoy Yourself. Make your program one that satisfies your soul along with your body. If you hate your program, chances are you won't stick with it.

Top Ten List for Injury Prevention

1. Optimize. Do the least workout that will maximize your capabilities.
2. Variety. Cross-train. Change routines that have repetitive forces.
3. Get enough rest.
4. Avoid errors in technique. It's estimated that about two-thirds of all injuries come from training errors.
5. Get good nutrition. Most people don't drink enough water. Drink more water.
6. Remember total body fitness. Train for strength, flexibility, and endurance of all your body.
7. If your resting pulse in the morning suddenly goes up more than 4 beats per minute over normal, that is a sign of overtraining.
8. Listen to your body. It has a lot of good things to say.
9. Alternate hard days with easy days.
10. Customize your program to suit your body, rather than copying an off-the-shelf program from a book or a trainer.

Source: Dr. Stanley L. James, University of Oregon, 1997 meeting of the American College of Sports Medicine.

What to Do When You've Already Done Too Much

Diagnose

You've done it. You're hurt. Go get a complete and accurate diagnosis of the injury, or injuries. There are usually more than one by this point. The key is not to treat until you know the cause, so that proper treatment may follow. Get an accurate diagnosis from a physician specializing in orthopedics. The Greek word *gnosis* means "knowing or recognizing." *Dia* is a word element that, in this context, means "completely." It's helpful to "completely know." Getting rid of pain and the disability that goes with it means treating the cause. Don't let any practitioner treat you without first knowing what's wrong. It is easy and effective, at the time, to treat the symptoms, but without knowing the cause, you can't change behavior and practices that will probably bring back the injury, and turn it into a chronic problem.

First Aid

Not discounting the importance of accurate diagnosis, many injuries take similar first aid. The first letters of the words rest, ice, compression, and elevation spell RICE, the acronym for treatment of almost all acute orthopedic injuries. Rest means rest. It doesn't mean exercising even if it hurts. It means letting yourself begin healing. It does include gentle range of motion and activity, according to your physician's instructions. It doesn't mean letting the rest of your body go to seed in the interim. Work other areas. Gradually get back to speed, always working below what it takes to reproduce the pain.

Use ice, not heat, for the first few days to reduce pain and swelling. You can continue to use ice even later if it helps to reduce pain. After about 48 hours, you can decide whether ice or heat is better for you. Until then, use ice. Bags of frozen peas or corn make good, pliant ice packs if no others are available. Physical therapist Marla Tonseth recommends freezing a mixture of one-third rubbing alcohol with two-thirds water in a zip lock bag to make a nice cool slush bag.

Compression with ace bandages reduces swelling in limb injuries. Elevation means elevating the injured part above your heart, not just propping it on a low chair. Antiinflammatory medications like aspirin or Motrin® help with pain and inflammation. Tylenol® has no antiinflammatory action but is good for pain if you can't stomach aspirin.

Stretch

Stretching helps alleviate delayed-onset soreness. Warm up gently, then just as gently, stretch the affected muscle slowly. A good place to stretch sore muscles is in a hot bath or shower. Don't stretch in a way that causes more pain.

What to Do When You've Already Done Too Much

First Aid. The first letters of the words *rest, ice, compression,* and *elevation* spell RICE, the acronym for treatment of many acute orthopedic injuries. Antiinflammatories help reduce pain and inflammation.

Diagnose. Get a complete and accurate diagnosis of the injuries.

Treat. Treat the cause of the injuries, not just the symptoms.

Stretch. Gentle stretching alleviates delayed onset soreness.

How to Do Without Overdoing

An exciting area of sports medicine research is devising screening and training programs that maximize physical potential without killing the exerciser. The amount and kind of exercise is different for everyone. Don't be dissuaded from exercise. It's much more common to rust out from inactivity than wear out from overdoing. Here are a few things to try:

Start Easy

For beginners, a twice-a-week program is often enough for the first months. Improvements in a previously sedentary or overweight person will be substantial. Weight loss occurs, waistlines shrink, fitness level and capacity for strenuous exercise improve, as does ability to tolerate heat and cold. Gains from twice-weekly programs occur more slowly than from exercise three or four days per week, but exercise is more likely to become part of a lifestyle, less likely to be skipped, with less chance of burnout.

Define Your Goals

Do you want to get stronger? Bigger? Smaller? The right exercises are different for each goal. *See* Chapters 2 and 3, "The Different Aspects of Fitness" and "Improving Your Fitness," and Chapter 8, "What Exercises Do You Need to Be Fit?" for more about the right workout for each desired effect.

Exercise Without Going to the Gym

Why ignore life by going to a gym all the time?

Make your daily activities your exercise. Take stairs instead of elevators; personally deliver messages instead of using interoffice mail; park farther away.

Make adventure your exercise. Take reconnaissance walks around your neighborhood. Carry packages for people. Help your local club lug things around. You might learn things, meet people, and work out all at once.

Make romance your exercise. You can walk in the park to feed geese as easily as going out to eat a fat dinner. Carry each other piggy back (observing good back mechanics). Walk all over town to find just the right flowers for a surprise. Walk to the post office often to mail frequent, friendly notes.

Remember the Rest of You

Your body is not the only part of you that needs exercise. Exercise your sensibilities. Exercise your smile muscles. Exercise your imagination. Exercise your funny bone. Exercise your love of life. Many things improve with exercise. Nice and easy.

How to Do Without Overdoing

Start Easy. For beginners, a twice-a-week program is often enough for the first several months. The gains occur more slowly than from exercising three or four days per week, but exercise is more likely to become part of a lifestyle, less likely to be skipped, with less chance of burnout.

Define Your Goals. Do you want to get stronger? Bigger? Smaller? The right exercises are different for each goal.

Exercise Without Going to the Gym. Make your daily work your exercise. Make having fun your exercise. Make romance your exercise. Why ignore life and mate by going to a gym all the time?

Remember the Rest of You. Exercise your sensibilities. Exercise your smile muscles. Exercise your imagination. Exercise your funny bone. Exercise your love of life.

11

Getting Out of Shape and How to Avoid It

We can now prove that large numbers of Americans are dying from sitting on their behinds.

—Bruce B. Dan

You may not be an exerciser. Or you may have started a program and got tired of it, or gone on vacation, or got caught up with work. You may have worked hard to get in shape at one time, but gave it up. After a layoff from exercise, your problems are more far-reaching than just gaining a little weight.

Loss of strength, endurance, and flexibility make packages seem heavier, runs longer, shelves harder to reach. Where did all those improvements you made go? Why should you care? What can you do?

How to Get Out of Shape

After long periods of not exercising, weights seem heavier than they used to. Following weeks of weightless space flight, astronauts come home with less muscle, blood volume, and bone than they left with. Even after only a day or two in bed with flu, you get up weak and dizzy even though you're not sick anymore. The principle of "Use it or lose it" is technically known as "reversibility." Physical performance gains made through exercise reverse with inactivity. The deterioration of your physical condition is technically known as *deconditioning*.

There are several ways to decondition. Just sitting around for the winter is one. Holiday gatherings and family obligations leave less time for the gym. Winter weather decreases routine outdoor excursions and recreational opportunities. These are technically known as "excuses."

Periods of inactivity often follow injury or illness. Deconditioning may be local as in a limb in a cast, or a global problem of whole body inactivity. The common mechanism is disuse. An immobilized limb dramatically decreases in size, strength, and endurance. Bed rest severely reduces the mechanical stresses your entire body needs to stay healthy. Bed rest so effectively deconditions you that aviation scientists use it to study physical decrements following zero gravity in space flight.

What Goes Bad?

Getting fat is only the tip of the pathologic iceberg of getting out of shape. Deconditioning seriously affects the functional state of your entire body. Strength, cardiovascular capacity, blood, mental skills, even your bones and immune system suffer.

Muscle

Without use, muscles decrease strength, endurance, and size, and lose blood vessel and nerve associations. They become less able to extract and use oxygen to do work, not only because your entire body's oxygen carrying and delivery system declines, but for chemical reasons of their own.

In-shape muscle is able to burn more fat as fuel than out-of-shape muscle, which uses more carbohydrate. Deconditioned muscles lose intracellular fluid, stored carbohydrate, and contractile protein, contributing to loss of muscle tone. Your body gets soft. Eating extra protein will not stop muscle protein loss. Only exercise does that. The bottom line is that when muscles decondition, you may not look as good, feel as good, exercise as much, or even do as much around the house.

Cardiovascular

A deconditioned cardiovascular system can't process, deliver, or burn enough oxygen to do intense exercise because several of its components go to seed with inactivity. The total amount of blood your heart pumps per minute decreases, probably from an overall decrease in blood volume in the initial weeks of detraining. You lose oxygen-carrying molecules called hemoglobin.

The size and contractile force of your heart diminishes. The maximum rate your heart can beat doesn't change, yet it has to beat faster and work harder to do the same work you could easily do when you were in better shape. More lactic acid builds up than if you weren't deconditioned. Cardiovascular deconditioning even lowers your ability to regulate body temperature in the heat and cold.

Bone

After your mid-thirties to forties, you usually begin losing bone if you don't exercise, no matter how much calcium you eat. To maintain mineral density, bones need the mechanical stress of muscles pulling on them. Bone loss is a major problem of space flight. As yet no countermeasures completely halt bone loss while weightless. On earth, sedentary lifestyle is a major risk factor for osteoporosis. Once osteoporosis develops, it is not reversible.

Body Composition

Although you may or may not avoid overeating during the winter holidays, without exercise you'll lose lean weight and put on some fat. Change in body composition over time includes higher body fat percentage and less lean muscle, even with no change in weight.

Cholesterol

One of several reasons regular exercise decreases risk of coronary artery disease is a favorable change in blood cholesterol. High-density lipoprotein cholesterol (HDL), popularly called good cholesterol, increases. "Bad cholesterol" or low-density lipoprotein (LDL) can decrease.

One study of male runners accustomed to 30–40 miles per week found detraining of only 2–3 weeks resulted in a 12% reduction in their aerobic capacity and a 7.7% reduction in good cholesterol. For more about good and bad cholesterol, see Part III.

Memory and Coordination

Sports skills not used over a winter dull and fade from active memory. Both memory and specific skills like fine motor coordination appear to involve physical and chemical connections that require practice to stay sharp.

Flexibility

Inactivity, not exercise, reduces flexibility. As joints tighten and your range of motion diminishes for normal, daily activities, you become more likely to pull or strain a muscle, particularly your back and hamstrings. Someone with tight, weak back muscles is a gear-bag accident waiting to happen. Weak, tight back and trunk muscles are the most usual cause of most back pain.

How Long Does It Take?

Even brief detraining periods remarkably reduce physical ability. After only days to weeks of stopping exercise, your capacity for exercise decreases. After longer periods of weeks to months, you can become a complete lump. Gains made from a summer in the gym and pool can disappear over a sedentary winter.

The more drastic your inactivity, the greater and more rapid your losses. Complete bed rest for a week can decrease your capacity to use oxygen, your strength, your hemoglobin count, and your blood volume by up to 7%. It would take several weeks to deteriorate to the same extent without bed rest even if you didn't exercise.

Does It Hurt?

In one sense you could say getting out of shape doesn't hurt. Deconditioning isn't physically painful. You won't even notice it's happening at first. The harm comes from the fact that getting out of shape is more serious than just gaining a little weight. The global physical decline not only hinders specific sport activities, but activities of daily living.

Capacity for routine walking, lifting, and carrying dwindles. You slowly weaken and as a result do less and push it less. In turn, you decondition further. A negative cycle self-perpetuates. Risk of cardiovascular disease, falls, back pain, obesity, musculotendinous strains, and certain cancers may increase. For these reasons you could say getting out of shape hurts a great deal.

In older people, deconditioning often continues to the point of severe and even dangerous weakness. Getting out of chairs and ordinary daily activities become too much. A serious handicap results, not from aging, but from preventable and reversible deconditioning.

These people, under physician supervision, benefit by regular weight lifting and conditioning programs. Several studies of exercise for populations debilitated by what we formerly called "aging" found dramatic reversals after simple weight lifting and activity programs. These people no longer needed canes or wheelchairs, decreased medications they took for high blood pressure, arthritis, or diabetes, and went back to unaided daily activities.

Preventing Getting out of Shape

At Least Do a Little

If you must take time off from exercise, try cutting back, not out. You can hold on to physical fitness even with less frequency of exercise if you maintain the intensity. According to some studies, cutting back from three regular days of exercise to two maintenance days can completely preserve oxygen-carrying capacity. Substituting one day for three will not prevent, but can reduce the consequences of detraining.

Avoid Bed Rest

In many instances, the original illness or injury is worsened through the physical degeneration resulting from bed rest. Sometimes irreversible problems develop. Current treatments for most illness and injury involve early ambulation.

Get Active, Stay Active

If you exercise, stay as active as you can all year every year. If you are sedentary, find some kind of regular activity you enjoy and get started. The older you get, the more beneficial exercise, including weight lifting, becomes. Exercise can at least partially counteract the physical deterioration of aging. A few table push-aways won't hurt either.

Stay in Shape

Getting out of shape is more serious than just gaining a little weight. It sabotages your cardiovascular condition, strength, endurance, bone health, blood fat status, body composition, and joint range of motion. In a short time, these decrements can become the functional equivalent of aging many years.

Serious problems can result from a vicious cycle of deconditioning, weakness, and poor health. This cycle is easily preventable. Staying in shape once you are active is easier than getting back in shape. You don't have to take care of your entire body, just the parts you want to keep.

12

Exercise Gimmicks

The actress Billie Burke was dining in a restaurant where, at the next table, a man was obviously suffering from a bad cold.

"I can see you're very uncomfortable," she volunteered. "So, I'll tell you what to do for it: drink lots of orange juice and take lots of aspirin. When you get to bed, cover yourself with as many blankets as you can find. Sweat the cold out. Believe me, I know what I'm talking about. I am Billie Burke of Hollywood."

The man smiled and introduced himself in return: "Thank you. I am Dr. Mayo of the Mayo Clinic."

It seems to be common for exercises to be taught, and health and fitness products promoted, by Hollywood stars and other self-proclaimed experts. Many humorous and outright wrong ideas and statements become commonly accepted:

Lose fat while you sleep by drinking miracle liquid, not available in stores.

Watch TV while motorized stomach vibrator burns more calories than 500 sit-ups a day.

Shrink your waist with secret device known for years to scuba divers.

You've probably seen these catchy ads via tabloids, magazines, and late-night television. Are they true? Yes. Is there a catch? Yes.

Regarding the first claim, everyone burns fat when they're asleep. When they're awake, too. Metabolizing stored fat is part of your round-the-clock energy production for body functions, whether you drink a "miracle liquid" or not. *See* Chapter 4, "What Does 'Aerobic' Really

Mean?," for more on the issue of fat burning, and Chapter 14, "Nutrition Myths," for more on how potions get sold by carefully worded, but false claims.

The second advertisement compares the relative number of calories burned in a longer time frame to a shorter one. In two hours sitting in front of the television wearing the device, you would burn more calories than during the theoretical 15–30 minutes it would take to do the sit-ups, with or without a vibrator strapped to your abdomen. That's just your normal metabolism at work.

Claims of Continued Fat Burning

Some products claim to give a workout so intense that you burn fat for hours after you finish. You burn fat 24 hours a day as part of being alive. It is also the case that during vigorous exercise, you increase your metabolism to meet your energy needs. Of course, it slows when you stop exercising, but takes a while to return to your resting values, sometimes up to a day. So any product can truthfully claim to produce increased calorie burning after a workout. A nice run or swim will do the same, although some evidence points to longer bouts of raised postexercise energy expenditure after resistance training than after aerobic exercise.

Aerobic Benefits by Just Increasing Heart Rate

Many activities like to promote themselves as beneficial for your cardiovascular system. Not everything that increases your heart rate or blood flow gives you aerobic benefits. For example, it is sometimes stated that the Yoga position of standing on the head or inclining head-down improves circulation and oxygenation to the head, and therefore confers aerobic benefit. Or that a specific stretch that is difficult to hold and raises heart rate therefore gives aerobic benefit. Neither improves aerobic capacity.

There is more to aerobic exercise than increasing blood flow and heart rate. Many things increase heart rate—for example, fear—without having anything to do with cardiovascular improvement. Increased heart rate from stage fright, for instance, is termed *neurogenic,* meaning it is produced as a nervous system effect, not *cardiogenic,* a cardiovascular system effect. Just moving the legs of a person lying in bed raises heart rate. It is a neurogenic increase, as that seems to be the body's way of preparing for exercise. Taking a long hot shower or sitting in a hot tub increases heart rate because your skin blood vessels open up to try to dump the extra heat from your body. The vasodilation lowers your blood pressure, and your heart usually must speed up to keep enough blood pumping around. There is no aerobic benefit to overheating. Even massage has been sometimes falsely promoted as beneficial to the cardiovascular system on the basis of increasing blood flow. That doesn't mean that massage is bogus or not helpful, just that it doesn't benefit your cardiovascular capacity. True aerobic benefit comes from a collection of effects that you can get only through long-duration exercise, repeated regularly over time.

Ab Isolators

There are several products on the market claiming to better isolate your abdominal muscles, and therefore somehow give you the same, spectacular abdomen as pictured on the package. The true way to get a trim, well-defined abdomen is to lower your body fat through long-term exercise, eat healthful meals on a regular basis, and do exercises to improve the size and shape of the abdominal muscles, whether you use an "isolator" or not. There is nothing in an isolating device that you cannot do without the device. For instance, the advertising for one device claims to hold your feet and legs in the specific position required for crunches. You can easily do that yourself without the device.

Other various devices on the market add resistance to the abdominal exercises. More resistance increases the muscle-unit activation you require to do the exercise, the same as carrying extra packages adds more weight to your arms. There is nothing secret or scientific about doing more work to get more results.

Dr. Steven Fleck, sport physiologist formerly with the U.S. Olympic Training Center, reminds us, "The value of these devices is their novelty. If they get you to exercise areas that you wouldn't normally exercise, they might pay for themselves." But remember that the fine print on the packaging mentions that these products need to be combined with healthy eating and regular exercise.

Secret Scuba Device

What is the secret scuba device mentioned in the beginning of this story? Neoprene. You've probably seen neoprene bands to wear around the waist and thighs. Yes, they shrink your waist, and yes it's another gimmick. It has nothing to do with sweat loss. Ever take off your socks? There's a darkened dent around your leg where the elastic compressed your flesh, leaving you temporarily smaller. You return to normal circumference soon enough. It's healthier, more economical, and longer lasting to just get in shape.

13

How to Get Started Getting in Shape

A man ought to have a doctor's prescription to be allowed to use a golf cart.

—Paul Dudley White

You know it's good for you, and you know you should get started. Some people are expert at starting an exercise program. They've done it hundreds of times. The trick is staying started.

Lifetime Activity

You don't have to go to a gym to get exercise. You don't have to do push-ups or jumping jacks, or run. You can develop fitness through an active lifestyle. Being active for fun, and for things you have to do anyway, is the concept of lifetime activity.

Your daily activities become more active in a natural way, instead of a sedentary life that has to be made up for by going to a gym. Shake up your concept of exercise from a hated mandatory session with strange rules about heart rates, intensities, and minimum calories to burn, into a daily life exercise playground—yard work, shopping, cleaning, painting. Make opportunities to burn calories as part of your normal daily routine. With a little imagination you could burn an extra 250–300 calories a day depending on your size. You'll lose 2–3 pounds a month. That may not sound like much but it's a clothing size every 3–4 months, and 20–30 pounds by next year.

Goal-Specific Exercise

Your plan of attack depends on your fitness goal. For a sedentary beginner to increase aerobic capacity, a three-times-a-week effort is a good starting place.

For disease reduction, three 10-minute walks a day can reduce your risk of early death by disease by 60 percent, according to the Cooper Institute for Aerobics Research in Dallas.

For fat reduction, start out with long low-intensity cardiovascular sessions and weight lifting. Weight lifting doesn't burn many calories during the workout, but increases your own lean weight, a helpful calorie burner. Food items are not worked off in single death-bouts. Small caloric expenditures multiply over time. A 150-calorie walk per day translates into just over 15 pounds a year. As with many other new physical activities, see your physician first.

Daily Fun, Not Specific Exercises

A key to getting fitter is finding activities you love to do, and make your daily routines more active in general. Some people want the same routine each day. Others need variety. But rather than think of fitness as intentional exercise at set periods for specific body parts, enjoy an active life. If you're heavy or haven't had a recent physical, see your physician before starting. Enjoy yourself. Don't overdo. Here are some ideas:

- Do you like to go dancing? Find a club and live it up weekly for a fun cardiovascular session.
- Walk to the market, carry home bags, and help put away groceries. That's both aerobic and muscular endurance, and depending on weight of the bags, some strength work, too.
- Try bicycling for errands or scenery for aerobic endurance and muscular endurance of the legs.
- Take nature walks.
- Plant a garden.
- Vacuum the house.

- Wash your car by hand and have fun getting your helpers all soapy.
- Take a walk and feed a few expired parking meters for strangers.
- Park farther away and walk the rest.
- Instead of swimming laps, play in the water with beach balls, foam floats, and kickboards.
- If you hate jogging, play Frisbee, tag, catch, or badminton instead. They may not always be as much exercise, but it is a way to get started and have fun.
- Why endure an impatient minute for an elevator when you can improve your legs on the stairs in half the time?
- If you work on a high floor, take the elevator a few flights and walk the rest.
- Hand-deliver interoffice mail.
- Help your local club or group with chores.
- Forget the golf cart and walk.
- Use a push mower instead of a power mower, a walk-behind mower instead of a ride-around mower.
- Hide the remote control.
- Give a friend a piggyback ride.
- Play with children.
- Be a hero and carry things for people.
- Take house-bound neighbor dogs for walks and romps.
- Walk-through instead of drive-through.
- Take reconnaissance walks all over your neighborhood. Drive to beautiful nature trails if none are close by, and take a walk.

SOME LIFESTYLE EXERCISES

Light Exercise: Less than 280 calories an hour	Moderate Exercise: 280–420 calories an hour	Vigorous Exercise: More than 420 calories an hour
Walking or strolling around 2 miles per hour	Fast walking: 3–4 miles per hour	Fast walking up a hill, or with a load
Golfing with a cart	Golfing carrying clubs	Racquet sports
Home care like vacuuming	House cleaning	Moving furniture
Mowing the lawn with a riding mower	Mowing the lawn with a power mower	Mowing the lawn with a push mower

Your Fitness Future

Make your daily life active and fun and you never have to go to a gym if you don't want to. Find activities you like to do anyway, and make them a part of your daily life. There are many things you will find that you like, or used to like, that would make your life better to add back into the day. Sit down and plan them out. Then get up and do them. Enjoy.

Part Two

Nutrition

How strange a creature is man, who will at times go to such extremes to preserve his life, only to shorten it at the dinner table.

—WILLIAM H. GORDON

14

Nutrition Myths

You believe easily that which you hope for earnestly.

—Terence (Greek-born Roman playwright, second century B.C.)

Nothing is so firmly believed as that which we least know.

—Michel de Montaigne (sixteenth-century French essayist)

If you heard of a nutrient your body requires to transmit nervous system signals, manufacture sex hormones, and is a precursor of the bile that handles ingested fats, would you eat lots of it?

It's cholesterol.

Would you run out and buy a substance your brain can't do without to process decisions and retain memory?

It's sugar.

Do you avoid a common practice using a chemical that constricts brain blood vessels, reducing cerebral blood flow?

It's breathing oxygen.

Descriptions in isolation can mislead. That's how nutrition myths begin. Ordinary food items become income producers to the slick packager. Nutrition myths are no exception. Here are just a few.

The "Isolated Aspect" Myth

Oxygen, in high concentrations, is toxic to every life form on the planet. If you breathe high levels for long periods, you will suffer ill effects. But you don't avoid breathing oxygen in the air around you. You use it for other characteristics in its favor, like staying alive. In similar ways, vitamin and food supplement advertisements divert your focus to and from isolated aspects of their product. They concentrate on problems occurring only from excesses or deficiencies, or on only one effect of the substance, usually exaggerated.

For Example, Here Are Two Claims:

A powdered carbohydrate supplement for weight lifters and athletes advertises that it is *insulinogenic*. The suffix *-gen* comes from a Greek word meaning "producing." In other words, it encourages insulin production. The advertising states that insulin is instrumental in getting the building blocks of protein into your muscle cells, and since this product is insulinogenic, it therefore builds muscle. Wouldn't that be great?

Another product uses exactly the opposite property of insulin for marketing. A popular high-protein diet promotes the idea that you must avoid nonprotein foods because they stimulate insulin. Since another property of insulin is to promote fat storage, these people say to eat only high-protein, non-insulin-stimulating foods, in order to be in a fat-burning "zone."

Here's the Critical Reading:

1. Insulin has several functions. It transports amino acids into your cells for protein synthesis. It also activates enzymes which stimu-late fat cells to synthesize and store fat. That's just part of how you digest food. So insulin helps you store fat. They don't say that on the labels for insulinogenic muscle-building supple-ments. They only tell you about storing protein, leading you to believe that their product will increase the normal amount of protein that you use to build your muscles. It doesn't.

2. Protein synthesis goes on all the time to replace the continual turnover in your cells. It doesn't construct a bigger muscle and bulge it through your skin (*see* "The 'More the Merrier' Myth," below, to understand why).

3. Almost all food is insulinogenic, particularly sugar. *Every* time sugar enters the nondiabetic bloodstream, it stimulates insulin release. There's nothing special about the "insulinogenic" prod-uct. It's just a sugary food.

4. The high-protein diet claims are misleading and potentially unhealthy. High-protein diets "work" to produce weight loss because they are low-calorie, not because of any insulin-stimulating or -suppressing quality.

The "More the Merrier" Myth

Most of your brain is water. Almost no one would expect to get more brain by drinking more water (I say "almost no one" with great optimism). If you eat an extra amount of something, your body doesn't always use it to do what you hope. Here's where the myths go wild. The most flagrant examples involve protein and calcium supplements.

By themselves, eating protein and taking calcium won't grow muscles or strengthen bones. Your body continually "turns over" the protein in muscle fibers, calcium in bone cells, and fat in fat cells. That means it uses some for body function, recycles some, and takes small amounts of incoming material from food for rebuilding. The constant breakdown and resynthesis is called modeling. Modeling doesn't grab extra protein or calcium and add it on to you. It takes what it needs to keep you the same as before and discards the rest, unless you give your body a reason to make you different than before. That reason is resistance exercise, also called weight lifting. Weight lifting will make your body add more protein to your muscles, and calcium to your bones. But just eating a food will not. For more on calcium and your bones, *see* Chapter 22 in Part III.

Another common place for the "More the Merrier" myth is vitamins. If a vitamin helps something in your body, then taking more vitamins must do more of that process? The B vitamins, for example, work as coenzymes. Coenzymes help an enzyme do its enzyme job. The enzyme/coenzyme interdependence is like a lock-and-key relationship. Only one key fits one companion lock. Taking more of a vitamin when your body is not making more of the corresponding enzyme will have no effect. From three wheels you can still make only one bicycle. Taking the companion enzyme in pill form will not help because eating the pills destroys the enzymes, described below in "The 'No Digestion' Myth."

Here's another example: A precursor of the bile that handles fat digestion is cholesterol. But if you eat more cholesterol, that won't make your body digest more fat. Your body uses what cholesterol it needs and dumps the rest back into your circulation. Too much cholesterol can have a tragic effect, bringing us to "The 'More Can't Hurt' Myth."

The "More Can't Hurt" Myth

Here's a Claim:

Protein builds muscles, therefore more protein must build more muscle, and after all, more can't hurt.

Here's the Critical Reading:

1. Extra protein doesn't build extra muscle unless plenty of resistance exercise tells your body that the muscle is needed.
2. Even then your body can only use so much, regardless of how much you exercise.
3. Past that amount, extra protein can harm.

Problems of Too Much Protein

Extra protein is not stored; it goes several routes. One is through your excretory system, taking water with it to produce urea. With excessive protein intake, you can dehydrate yourself a bit. Another exit route for excess protein is conversion to fat, which can't be turned back to protein later. Another problem with too much protein is that it increases calcium loss through the urine. That means that eating too much protein makes you "pee" out calcium. Epidemiologic studies point to excess protein, particularly animal protein, as contributing to osteoporosis.

What about those high-protein diets that claim you need extra protein to get you into a fat-burning zone? It turns out that if you follow their meal plans, the meals are low-calorie, and for that reason, you lose weight. It does not have anything to do with extra protein, or insulin, or zones. Problems occur because the meals are also low-carbohydrate, which leaves you tired. You need energy to carry out daily activities, and to exercise for weight loss and health you do need a certain amount of protein every day. Chapter 18 covers the details to figure out how much you will need.

Problems of Too Much Iron

Blood iron level is another thing frequently thought to be better with more than less. That is not always true. Iron is essential to your health, in several roles. Iron is also involved in certain harmful reactions in your body, involving special molecules called free radicals (for more on free radicals see the glossary, and below in the sections on "The 'No Digestion' Myth" and "The 'Reverse Reasoning' Myth"). Free radicals can sometimes be very destructive in your body. That's their job. People with high iron have been found to develop high rates of heart disease, possibly from high amounts of free radicals generated from too much iron. Although women are frequently labeled as at a disadvantage for their tendency to have lower iron levels than men, it seems that may have developed to be an advantage. Populations with lower than average iron levels have been found to have lower than average incidence of heart disease. Iron is only one of many factors, not the only factor involved in this phenomenon, but it is not an unimportant consideration. *See* Chapter 27, "Cardiovascular Disease," for more about the possible connection between too much iron and heart trouble. If that weren't enough, iron supplements are constipating. It is now a common recommendation that people should not supplement iron without physician supervision.

Even Water

Even drinking water can be overdone. It's not common, but extreme, prolonged exercise in the heat, with no food or fluid replacement other than large amounts of water, can cause a problem called water intoxication. You just dilute yourself too much.

More is not always better. Philosopher Allen Ross Anderson capsulized maximalist thinking: "We should have our minds open, but not so open that our brains fall out."

The "No Digestion" Myth

More is not always better. Sometimes more becomes nothing at all. Some health food stores sell pills containing enzymes. The claims are that your body needs these enzymes for various functions, so if you take a supply of these enzymes in their pills, you will get more of the benefits. This does not work at all.

First, there is no way for enzymes to get into your bloodstream by ingesting them. They cannot pass through your intestinal wall except by breaking down into constituent parts. This destroys them as enzymes.

Broken-down enzymes will not automatically reassemble on the other side of your intestine, so eating enzymes will not raise your body levels of enzymes. Your body makes all the enzymes you need out of the ordinary food you eat. Eating enzymes by themselves, except those that aid digestion like lactase to digest dairy products, is useless and expensive.

An interesting example is superoxide dismutase (SOD). SOD is an enzyme that is one of several antioxidants your body needs and makes to counter the effects of free radicals, which are generally accepted as being a cause of many physical problems.

Free radicals have an unpaired electron, so they go around trying to get another electron for themselves by taking one from other molecules in your body. Free radicals particularly target fatty acids and proteins, harming them in the process of stealing their electrons. Then the fatty acids and proteins become free radicals themselves, and go around grabbing electrons from other molecules, like a destructive game of tag. Your body has several built-in systems for removing radicals, but can get overwhelmed by too many free radicals, which can then go unchecked in their damage.

Eating SOD in pill form won't do anything against free radical damage or any other oxidative stress in your body. If eaten, SOD, like any other enzyme, is destroyed in your intestine by digestion.

As is often the case with sham cures offered in pill form, there are many research studies that seem to back up the claims. Studies do show that SOD reduces free radical formation. None of these studies involved eating the SOD, but injecting it into laboratory animals under specific conditions. More on free radicals, oxygen toxicity, and antioxidants below in "The 'Reverse Reasoning' Myth."

The "It Works for Popeye" Myth

People frequently want to know if a food or sports bar advertised as "giving energy" really will perk them up. These products are just food, not stimulant drugs such as cocaine or amphetamines. However, many do contain stimulants such as caffeine, ginseng, ma huang, or other substances explained in Chapter 17, "Ergogenic Aids."

Technically, the potential energy in food is measured in units called calories. "High-energy snack" is a euphemism for "high-calorie food" or, in other words, "fattening food." If you eat high quantities of high-energy food, it really will give you potential chemical energy for your activities right now, and plenty more for the future. That stored energy is called fat. Armed with this knowledge, you can now pick out the person who obviously has the most energy at hand (and other places) for activities—an obese person.

What About Vitamins?

Vitamins have no calories so, technically, furnish no energy. If you are vitamin deficient in a way that makes you weak, then restoring healthy levels will restore your normal energy levels. Extra vitamins will not give you "pep." More on vitamins in "The 'Reverse Reasoning' Myth."

What About Sugar?

Sugar makes you feel energetic shortly after eating it. Sugar helps delay fatigue if used during long endurance events where you can't stop to eat. Simple sugars make your insulin levels soar to deal with the sugar, then drop soon after, making you feel tired. That's the problem with eating sugar for energy. Complex sugars (complex carbohydrates) have a steadying effect on insulin, and are a better choice for eating for energy. Regularly relying on simple sugars for "quick fixes" is not the healthiest choice. Although a complex topic, the main idea is to eat smaller, more frequent, low-fat, high-complex carbohydrate meals every day, and do the work that increases your musculature and fitness. Then you are capable of more energy for exercise. Regular good nutrition and regular exercise, not special energy foods, give you energy.

Claims of enhanced athletic performance and energy from health foods, supplements, vitamins, steroids, caffeine, amphetamines, and others are examined in Chapter 17.

The "Need It Now" Myth

People sometimes ask which vitamins and minerals that sporting activities take out of your system, and which specific foods have those nutrients, so that they can eat them before exercise. General recreational exercise does not sufficiently deplete any nutrients to affect athletic ability or health. For that reason, after a one-hour hike or game of tennis you don't need to immediately replace specific vitamins or minerals. Your next good meal will cover you. It is unnecessary to take extra vitamins or minerals ahead of time to offset any loss predicted during your exercise. You don't lose enough to affect performance or fatigue level. Regular healthy eating and hydration assures you don't start your day in an already depleted state. Moreover, your daily requirements of most nutrients typically balance out over days. Minute-to-minute deficits don't matter as much. Drinking water is always a good idea before and after exercise.

Here's a Claim:

It's often said you are in danger of B_{12} deficiency if you don't eat red meat every day to make up the amounts you use every day.

Here's the Critical Reading:

A small number of people can't use the B_{12} in their diets. These people must take supplements or get injections. Otherwise, Vitamin B^{12} is stored in your liver in enormous quantities, sufficient for a three-to-five-year period.

The "Reverse Reasoning" Myth

If a deficit causes a weakness, a much-cherished myth is that a surplus will bring strength. But just as the right glasses prescription helps you see better, getting too strong a correction will not make you see even better.

Vitamin E is a good example. A while back, on experiments with rats, researchers removed all Vitamin E from the rat's diet. The rats became bald and sterile. Restoring Vitamin E restored the rat's hair and fertility. Human marketeers got hold of those results, and launched a very successful campaign to sell Vitamin E with claims of giving you hair and virility. Of course, Vitamin E does not do that for humans with adequate nutrition. (But bald, sterile rats, take note.)

Here Are Some Claims:

1. Vitamin A is often promoted as "Needed for good night vision."
2. High-calorie foods are often labeled as "Giving you energy."
3. Special powdered mixtures are advertised as "Providing all the nutrients contained in healthy spinal discs," or containing "All the nutrients crucial to healthy hair."
4. Free radicals are accepted to be involved in the various damage to the body caused by their highly oxidative nature. Vitamins C and E are known antioxidant agents against the oxidative free radical activity. People often take extra Vitamins C and E on the presumption that it will reduce their risk of the various damaging effects of free radicals.

Here's the Critical Reading:

1. Vitamin A deficiency reduces ability to see in dim light. But no amount of carrots or Vitamin A supplements will make adequately nourished eyes see better.
2. Calorie deficiency makes you tired. But eating extra calories will not make you energetic, it will make you fat.
3. Potions containing the nutrients or component substances of your back and hair don't fix your bad back or grow hair. They're regular food. Countless products line the shelves, truthfully stating they are for skin, nerves, strength, fingernails, or whatever— all just glamorized food. Yes, your body needs specific nutrients to do its job, but eating more of them won't increase the processes.
4. Vitamin E is lipid (fat) soluble and protects cell membranes, which have a major lipid component. Vitamin C is a water-soluble antioxidant, having protective effects in blood and the fluid inside and outside of cells. Vitamins E and C work together in their free radical inactivation work. The way Vitamin E inactivates radicals is to accept the extra electron that makes the molecules radical and reactive. When Vitamin E takes that extra electron, it becomes itself radical. Vitamin C then takes the extra electron from E to restore Vitamin E. Vitamin C is special, in that it can accept this extra burden without injury to itself or surrounding molecules.

You need a minimum amount of these vitamins to do their jobs. It's true that many people, particularly those on the typical meat heavy

Western diet, may not get enough Vitamins E and C, which are found in vegetables and fruits. But taking more Vitamins E and C than you need has not been shown to increase their usual effects on radicals in the body. If you are vitamin deficient, they may help, but not if you are vitamin sufficient. Taking too much can be injurious.

As an important note, free radicals are not all bad. There are some that perform critically important functions in your body, such as those involved in muscle contraction and in the immune response. You may not want to push your resting levels down, even if it were possible to do so by eating antioxidants. If you got rid of the radicals stored in special cells in your body that fight infection, you will be at serious risk of catastrophic infections.

The bottom line is that eating extra of any particular nutrient will not give you extra abilities. Although protein is a building block of your skin, eating extra protein will not make you grow lots of extra skin. Your body does not use the extra.

The "I Can Eat Anything I Want as Long as It Is Low-Fat" Myth

Eating low-fat and still not losing weight? Forget all the conflicting and confusing articles you've read about needing to eat fat for "zones" or fat burning, or that carbohydrates make you fat. It is the number of calories you eat of those "low-fat" foods that makes the difference. Low-fat cakes, cookies, and candies can easily be high-calorie and full of sugar. Obviously, an entire sack of sugar is nonfat (and a 1,000-calorie block of butter is "sugar-free," too). Keep your common sense about you. Several hundred extra calories a day of nonfat food will just be stored as fat.

The "I Eat Right" Myth

An average person sits down to an evening meal of steak or burgers, potato mashed with butter, salt, and milk, coffee with cream and sugar, a small side of buttered vegetables, then ice cream and/or cake for dessert. A good dinner of protein for muscles, calcium for bones, and energy for exercise? No. The U.S. Department of Agriculture recently surveyed American dietary habits. The findings? Many Americans who think they eat healthy don't at all. The sample dinner is typical of three times too much fat, saturated fat, cholesterol, and salt; double the needed protein; too much simple sugar; hardly any fiber, vitamins, or complex carbohydrates; and not enough water. This kind of eating is increasingly associated with heart and vascular disease, vitamin deficiency, dehydration, calcium loss, high blood pressure, and some cancers.

The "Healthy Eating Is Awful" Myth

Why should low-fat, vegetable-based meals be called drastic, while cardiac bypass surgery, stroke, and colon cancer are considered normal? This is good news not bad. Good meals need no secret energy foods and no special supplements. They can be delicious and healthy in many ways. What to eat is covered more comprehensively in Chapter 18, "Healthy Eating."

Escaping Myths

Some nutrition myths don't matter—stomachs don't digest food, that's the job of the small intestine. Some myths stem from mistaken identity—stomachs don't growl, that's the small intestine again. And some myths were just created to sell a product—there never was a real Betty Crocker. Food myths are sometimes like food itself. No matter how thin you slice it, it's still baloney.

15

Calculating Food Fat

I had fried mozzarella cheese. Deep-fried cheese. Oh, there's a cardiovascular dream come true. The cheese doesn't have enough fat—let's give it a cholesterol Jacuzzi!

—Rick Corso

You've been good. You've learned about good eating habits. You're making positive lifestyle changes. You eat less fat because that's how to get slimmer and healthier.

You even eat healthy in restaurants. You order salad with dressing on the side, vegetable soup, a potato (no bacon) that you plan to season with lemon-pepper, nonfat dressing, and spices, and spaghetti with spiced red sauce, no Parmesan.

The soup arrives cooked in a beef fat base, thickened with cream, topped with cheese. The potato arrives with a dip of sour cream, cheese, and butter. The entree was cooked with butter or oil. The red sauce is thickened with oil, corn starch, and flour.

The American Heart Association recommends no more than 30% of the calories you eat come from fat. The meal you thought you ordered would have totaled 735 calories including 185 calories of fat, or about 25% of the calories from fat, and would have been a good-tasting, healthy, low-fat meal. If you used seasonings instead of dressing, there would have been a mere 50 calories of fat out of 535 total, only 8.5% fat. What you got instead was a 1,558-calorie lunch, with 935 of those calories from fat, or 60% fat. Meanwhile, you thought you were eating low fat, and don't understand why the weight is so hard to keep off.

What You Thought You Ordered:

Item	Total Calories Low-Fat Version	% Fat Low-Fat Version
Salad	50	trace
Thousand Island dressing	150	86%
Vegetable soup	90	10%
Plain potato	145	5%
Spaghetti—no oil	200	4%
Low-fat sauce	100	27%

Total Calories: 735, or 585 without the salad dressing
Fat Calories: 185, or only 50 without the salad dressing
Percent Fat: 25%, or 8.5% without the salad dressing

What You Might Get Instead:

Item	Total Calories High-Fat Version	% Fat High-Fat Version
Salad	50	4%
Thousand Island dressing	150	87%
Creamed soup with cheese	322	45%
Potato with toppings	436	52%
Spaghetti in butter	300	38%
High-fat sauce	300	60%

Total Calories: 1,558
Fat Calories: 935
Percent Fat: 60%

How To Calculate Food Fat

How do you know if a food is high fat? If it has the words *fried, buttered,* or *rich* in the name, that's one clue. If you put the food on a napkin and it leaves the napkin transparent, that's another.

For most foods you won't know without looking on the label. The label tells many things, including how many calories and how many grams of fat are in the food. If the label doesn't state the fat percentage, calculating it is not hard. Divide the calories of fat by the total number of calories. If a food has 100 calories and 27 calories come from fat, the food is 27% fat.

To find how many calories of fat there are, multiply the number of grams of fat by 9. Why 9? There are 9 calories in each gram of fat. By comparison, there are 4 calories per gram of protein or carbohydrate.

To Calculate Percentage Fat In Any Food:

1. Find the number of grams of fat in the food.
2. Multiply the number of grams of fat by 9 to get calories of fat.
3. Find the total number of calories in the food.
4. Divide calories of fat (#2) by the total number of calories (#3).

How Much Fat?

Two main ways to keep track of the fat you eat are by grams and by percent. The result of each is the same. The method you choose is just a matter of personal preference.

The Percent Method

In the percent method you try to eat no more than a predefined percent of your daily calories as fat calories. The often-quoted maximum by the American Heart Association is 30%. Other organizations opt for lower percentages, including 10% fat diets that have a track record of being able to reverse cardiovascular disease. Learn the amount of fat contained in foods you eat and cut back on those with a high percentage.

The Gram Method

In the gram method, you track how many grams of fat you eat per day, and decide not to go over a certain number of grams per day.

To know how many grams of fat is right for you, you first need to know how many calories you need every day, then decide what percentage of that you will allow for fat. That tells you how many calories of fat you can have each day. Divide your total calorie need by 9 to find the maximum number of grams of fat. A sample calculation looks like this:

Calorie needs for average women are roughly 2,000-2,300, and for average men, 2,500 to 2,800 calories per day. These numbers change with activity and body size. If you decide that you will allow 30% of those calories as fat, it's 600–690 for women and 750–840 for men. Dividing by 9 to find the number of grams of fat would be 66–76 for women and 83–93 for men.

A rough estimate for the gram method, but without all the math, is to divide your body weight in pounds, or the weight you wish you were, by half. If you weigh 120 pounds (54 kilograms), you can have 60 grams. If you weigh 140 pounds (64 kilograms), you can have 70 grams. If you weigh 160 pounds (73 kilograms), you can have 80 grams. If you weigh 180 (82 kilograms), you can have 90 grams. If you weigh 200 pounds (91 kilograms), then 100 grams of fat per day will pretty much keep you at that weight. Reduce the grams of fat to reduce your fat intake.

If all of this seems too arcane, remember that you are still adding up just one thing—total fat in your diet. Clever advertising about percent fat, by weight, or any other claim that may appear on the back of the package, can be ignored. All you need to do is figure out how much of what you want to eat, and add it up.

Why 2% Milk Is Not 98% Fat Free

Food marketers want you to buy their product. Food labels often state the food is a certain percent "fat-free." Often that is misleading advertising.

What's important to your health is the percentage of total calories that come from fat. Advertisers often measure the fat by its weight in the product, which is meaningless to you and watching fat. A cup of "2% fat" milk is not 2% fat by calories. A surprising 35% of the total calories are from fat. Here's why.

One cup of 2% fat milk has 121 calories and 4.7 grams fat. Multiply the 9 calories per gram of fat by the number of grams, in this case 9

× 4.7 or 42.3. So 42.3 calories out of the total of 121 calories are from fat. Divide 42.3 by 121 to get 0.35. One cup of 2% fat milk is 35% fat.

Let's try one cup of whole milk, called 3% milk. It has 150 calories and 8 grams fat. Multiply 9 times 8 to get 72. Divide 72 by 150 to learn that whole milk is 48% fat.

What about one cup of 1% fat milk, which is labeled low-fat milk. It has 102 calories and 2.6 grams of fat. Nine times 2.6 is 23.4 calories of fat. Divide 23.4 by 102 to see that 1% fat milk is really 23% fat.

Now try one cup of skim milk, called nonfat milk. It has 86 calories and 0.5 grams of fat. Nine times 0.5 is 4.5 calories of fat out of 86 total. You can see that this is finally low fat—only 5% fat.

HOW LOW FAT IS LOW-FAT MILK?

Milk Product 8 ounces	Total Calories	Grams of Fat	Calories of Fat (grams × 9)	% Fat (calories of fat divided by total calories)
Whole milk 3%	150	8.0	72.0	72/150=48%
2% fat milk	121	4.7	42.3	35%
1% fat milk	102	2.6	23.4	23%
Skim milk	86	0.5	4.5	5%

(some figures rounded)

The Fat in Your Foods

The next chart tells about five popular meals. Just like the previous chart, the second column of the chart indicates the total number of calories. The third column tells grams of fat. Multiply the number of grams by 9 to know how many calories from each item come from fat, indicated in column 4. Divide by the total calories to get the percent of the calories that are fat, as shown in the last column.

Percentage Fat Is Not the Whole Story

A Big Mac and a croissant/egg/cheese/ham sandwich have nearly the same number of grams of fat. The greater number of calories in the Big Mac drops the percent fat to a deceptively lower figure, while not making the Big Mac the healthier choice. A serving of French fries has nearly the same number of calories as a bowl of pasta and broccoli. French fries have more than eight times more fat. A meal of pasta and broccoli has an amazing 5% or so of fat. A pack of fries—more than 40%.

HOW LOW FAT ARE COMMON FOODS?

Meal	Total Calories	Grams of Fat	Calories of Fat (grams × · 9)	% Fat (calories of fat divided by total calories)
Croissant/egg Cheese/ham	475	33.6	302.4	65%
Big Mac	560	33.0	297.0	53%
French fries	220	10.0	90.0	41%
Bowl of oatmeal with cinnamon	145	2.3	20.7	14%
Bowl of pasta and broccoli	223	1.2	10.8	<5%

(some figures rounded)

What About Dessert?

The chart below gives information about five popular desserts. The second column indicates the total number of calories. The third tells grams of fat. Multiply the number of grams by 9 to find out how many calories from that particular dessert are from fat. Then divide by the total to get the percentage of calories that are from fat.

HOW LOW FAT ARE FROZEN DESSERTS?

Dessert (greatly varies depending on brand)	Total Calories	Grams of Fat	Calories of Fat (grams × 9)	% Fat (calories of fat divided by total calories)
Ice cream (premium brand)	349	24	216	62%
Ice milk	184	6	54	29%
Frozen yogurt	180	4	36	20%
Sherbet	270	4	36	13%

(some figures rounded)

How Low Fat Are Movie Foods?

Movie Food	Total Calories	Grams of Fat	Calories of Fat (grams × 9)	% Fat (calories of fat divided by total calories)
Reese's Peanut Butter Cups (2)	250	15	135	54%
Small bag of M& Ms with peanuts	250	13	117	46.8%
Popcorn (2 cups)	80	4	36	45%
Small bag of M& Ms plain	230	10	90	39%
Box of Cracker Jack	120	3	27	22.5%
Air-popped popcorn (2 cups)	50	trace	trace	<<1%

(some figures rounded)

Snacks

Modern snack foods are loaded with fat. Drinking diet soda with high-fat snacks does not cancel out the calories. The following chart reflects some realistic quantities like handfuls, bars, and small bag-fulls, instead of the commonly listed serving sizes.

How Low Fat Are Snacks?

Snack	Total Calories	Grams of Fat	Calories of Fat (grams × 9)	% Fat (calories of fat divided by total calories)
Potato chips	316	21.8	196.2	62%
Fritos Corn Wild Mild Chips	150	9.0	81.0	54%
Almond Joy	250	14.0	126.0	50%
Snickers Bar	280	13.0	117.0	42%
Hard pretzels	212	3.5	31.5	15%
Bagel	163	1.4	12.6	8%
Banana	105	0.5	4.5	4%
Handful of raisins	65	trace	trace	<1%

(some figures rounded)

What if you added nonfat but high-calorie candy to a
snack of potato chips? Would that lower the figure for
total fat percentage compared to total calories?
Yes, it would. But that will not make that snack a healthier
one. You only added more calories and more simple
sugars. Total calories still count.

Meat

Many people regard meat as only a protein food, forgetting that
meat is usually a high-fat item.

How Low Fat Are Common Meats?

Meat	Total Calories	Grams of Fat	Calories of Fat (grams × 9)	% Fat (calories of fat divided by total calories)
Meat stick, smoked, 1 oz.	156.1	14.0	126.3	81%
Bacon, 2 slices	72.6	6.5	56	77%
Bologna, pork, 1 slice	56.8	4.6	41	72%
Pork chop, 1	284	22.3	201	70%
Salami, cooked, beef, 1 slice	60.3	4.8	43	70%
Hamburger, 1, baked, not fried	244	17.8	160	70%
Chicken, dark meat with skin, 3 oz.	215.4	13.5	122	60%
Ham, 1 slice	40	2.3	21	52%
Meat Loaf, frozen dinner	112.3	6.5	58	52%
Hot dog, 1 plain with the bun	242	14.5	130.5	50%
Chicken, light meat no skin, 3 oz. serving	147	3.8	34.5	23.5%
Turkey, dark meat, no skin	262	10	90	34%
Turkey, light meat, no skin	219	4.5	40.5	18%

(some figures rounded)

Now compare the calories and fat in the meats above to some imitation meats below. These vegetable "meats" can taste surprisingly like the real thing, and are also high in protein.

How Much Fat Is In Common Meat Substitutes?

Meat made from vegetable sources	Total Calories	Grams of Fat	Calories of Fat (grams × 9)	% Fat (calories of fat divided by total calories)
Green Giant Harvest Burger	140	4	36	26%
Fantastic Foods Nature's Burger	120	2	18	15%
Morningstar Farms Better'n Burgers	70	0	0	0%
Light Life Smart Dogs	45	0	0	0%

Simple Tips to Cut Back Fats

- Try oatmeal or other cereal for breakfast instead of croissants or Danish, and trade the Big Mac for a plate of pasta and broccoli for lunch or dinner. In one day you can drop from 60% fat to less than 10% for the two meals combined.
- High-fat foods like peanut butter and cake frosting licked off knives and spoons still count. Don't forget them when figuring your totals.
- Cutting out the two tablespoons of thousand island dressing in the sample lunch listed at the beginning of this chapter drops a 27% fat meal to 9%. If you can't do without dressing, use less—one tablespoon instead of two, or try low- or nonfat substitutes or seasonings and lemon instead of dressing.
- Many types of meat are usually far above the American Heart Association's recommended fat maximum. Cutting back on these will greatly reduce your daily fat intake.
- List your favorite foods. Find out how much fat is in each. See how many of the foods you like are low fat. Eat those.
- If you starve yourself, you will not be happy or healthy. Eventually you will probably rebound into the gooiest, fattiest foods you can find. Have healthy snacks when you are hungry.

- When making omelets, leave out a few (or most) of the egg yolks.
- Avoid eating too many high-sugar, high-calorie items that advertise as low fat. The sugar calories will creep up on you.
- Pastas are usually good bets, as are most vegetable dishes, but that depends on how much oil, cream, and butter you add.
- Don't panic if you eat one high-fat food. What counts is your long-term day in–day out consumption.
- Try more fruit and less pie to satisfy your sweet tooth. Make your own desserts, including low-fat recipes for pie. They will still be delicious.
- Even if no one sees you when you eat high-fat food, it still counts.

Resources for Keeping Track of Food Fat

Besides keeping track of food fat in your own notebook, one easy-to-use, well-organized book is the *Low Fat Diary* by Corinne T. Netzer, published by Dell Publishing. It is around $6.95 and has daily pages for recording meals and an index with a good list of fat grams in common foods.

16

Sport Drinks

Life is thirst.—Leonard Michaels

Dehydration is a common, but rarely recognized factor in fatigue. Dehydration greatly reduces your capacity for exercise and your tolerance to heat. Many sport drinks on the market claim to prevent dehydration better than plain water. Is that so? Sport drinks also state they replace electrolytes. What is an electrolyte and why and when do you need to replace them? What do these drinks really do?

What Are Sport Drinks?

You lose water and salts in normal processes all day. You also use up carbohydrates for energy. You need to replace what you lose. The first drink to bring all the needed ingredients together in one package was developed at the University of Florida, and named Gatorade® for their Gators mascot. The drink originally was used to replace fluids and carbohydrate energy during long exercise bouts. Now a variety of sport drinks in many different formulas are available for a variety of uses.

What Do Sport Drinks Do That Plain Water Doesn't?

Studies of exercise in the heat show that people prefer the taste of a salty drink, so they drink more. The bit of salt in these drinks stimulates thirst, then makes you retain the water you drink. The sugar content in sport drinks allows more water absorption through the intestine than from a solution of only salts. In other words, the sugar aids water absorption, helping replace needed water into your bloodstream. The sugar also supplies calories for exercise. Specially formulated "replacement drinks" have high carbohydrate amounts specifically for the purpose of restoring carbohydrates after exercise. The specifics on "carbo-loader" and "carbo-replacements" drinks are explained in Chapter 17 "Ergogenic Aids."

What Sport Drinks Do

- Increase palatability, compared to plain water, so you drink more.
- Replace needed water, then help absorb and retain water.
- Stimulate your thirst mechanism to keep you drinking.
- Provide carbohydrate during long exercise bouts to delay fatigue.
- Replace carbohydrate after exercise.

You Get Thirsty Two Ways

One way you get thirsty is when you are low on water, called hypovolemic thirst. If you replace only water, your body sees that you have more fluid relative to electrolytes, because you have also lost electrolytes. Your body helpfully responds by "peeing" out some water to balance things out. You may still be a bit low on water because of this, even after drinking water. The second way you get thirsty is when you have a high electrolyte blood content, regardless of your body's total water volume. This is called osmotic thirst. That is why salty things make you thirsty, even when you are drinking (and why bars serve you salty finger food—to keep you drinking). Small amounts of sodium in electrolyte drinks stimulate your osmotic thirst, then help you retain what you drink. That is why people drink more of these beverages than plain water.

What Is an Electrolyte Anyway?

An electrolyte is a substance that, when you dissolve it in liquid, becomes electrically conductive. Why does your body need an electric current? To transmit every signal for all the thousands of functions that nerves control to keep you alive, moving, and thinking, and to maintain an electrical potential across the member of every cell in your body, so that the cells can do their jobs.

No current flows through pure water. Dissolving even a trace of electrolytes in water makes water conductive. Electrolytes that are put into a liquid break up into ions. Ions are atoms or molecules with at least one electron fewer or more than normal, giving them a positive or negative electric charge. Table salt, for example, becomes the positively charged sodium ion, and the negatively charged chloride ion. Both are principal ions in your body. In physiology, the ions themselves are called electrolytes. Salt, itself, is not an electrolyte, but in liquid it becomes the ions that are electrolytes.

Flashlights run on current passed by electrons through wire.
Your body runs on current passed by ions through nerves.

The difference between current in electronic equipment and in your body is that electronic signals race through wire passed by electrons at up to half the speed of light, while in your body nerve signals move through ions thousands of times more slowly. Current in electronics uses electrons to pass the charge. The electrons themselves don't move far, but pass the charge along from one electron to the next like toppling dominos. In your body, nerve signals move along dissolved ions. Like electrons, the ions themselves don't move far in the nerve, but propagate the signal by positive and negative ions switching places on either side of the nerve membrane. That makes neighboring positive and negative ions want to switch places too, in a continuing action called the action potential, until the signal is passed along the nerve. Then the nerve ending uses a transmitter chemical to jump to the next nerve to start the signal traveling again, until the message is delivered.

Why Replace Electrolytes?

Losing some electrolytes through sweat is a good thing, to an extent. If you lost only water, your blood would get far too concentrated with electrolytes. Even though you lose electrolytes, your body regulates the loss so you don't lose too much. So, when you sweat, you lose proportionately more water than minerals, leaving your blood slightly more concentrated than normal, or hypertonic. Even though your body does not want to be more concentrated with electrolytes, that does not mean you should avoid drinks containing electrolytes. You can lose a substantial amount of electrolytes with prolonged sweating, creating a real need for replacement. Without replacement, your electrolyte and fluid levels fall too low, and your ability to exercise decreases. With extreme electrolyte loss during long exercise, and only water to drink, you may abnormally dilute your body fluids and cells, a condition called water intoxication. Effects range from weakness to convulsion and occasionally death. Water intoxication is also called hyponatremia (high-poe-nay-TREE'-me-uh), meaning low sodium in the blood. Cases are usually reported in hikers and distance runners who drink only large amounts of water and eat no food. Occasionally, serious cases of hyponatremia occur in infants swallowing pool water during parent-infant swimming lessons.

Your Body Regulates Electrolytes

You eat varying amounts of electrolytes in your food and drink, and lose varying amounts with exercise and daily activity. Your body ordinarily keeps levels of everything within narrow ranges, no matter how much you vary input and output. Your body restricts electrolyte loss when your supply is low, and gets rid of excess when you eat or drink too much. When you are inactive, the major exit avenue for surplus electrolytes is urine and feces. When you are active and start sweating more, your body restricts the amount of electrolytes that exits with sweat, and secretes a hormone called aldosterone (al-DOHS-tur-own) into your bloodstream to help your kidneys retain more sodium. Most people in Western society eat many times more salt than their bodies require, sometimes in astounding quantities in fast foods, and that's before they even pick up the salt shaker. When you eat more salt than you need, your body retains water to dilute the salt, and aldosterone secretion drops, encouraging your kidneys to excrete the excess. Ordinarily, your body handles large ranges of excess.

Some "salt-sensitive" people with high blood pressure need to restrict salt, to allow them to lose the extra water that salt retains. For the rest of the population, salt seems not to matter much. Your kidneys tightly regulate your output to get rid of excess electrolytes and water, or hang on to them depending on what you need at the time.

Many people worry about limiting salt intake. A small portion of the population is "salt-sensitive," and needs to restrict salt. For most other people however, the body takes care of eliminating excess.

When Should You Replace Electrolytes?

Except for extreme endurance activities, you usually eat and drink more than enough electrolytes with your regular meals to keep you going. Ordinary recreational exercise does not deplete electrolytes enough to affect athletic ability or health. For that reason, after a one-hour bout of exercise, you don't ordinarily need to replace electrolytes immediately. It is also unnecessary to take extra electrolytes ahead of time to offset any loss predicted during your short bout of exercise. You don't lose enough to affect performance or cause fatigue. Unless you are in endurance races, or work long hours in hot environments with limited chance to eat and drink fluids other than water, health problems from electrolyte loss is unlikely.

Do You Need Sport Drinks?

- If you do endurance events lasting more than an hour or so, like marathons and triathlons.
- If you exercise in the heat for long periods.
- If you like to drink semisweet drinks more than you like to drink water.

Why You Get Dehydrated from Drinking Sea Water

Seagoing birds such as penguins, seagulls, petrels, and albatross can drink sea water. Special glands in their heads excrete excess salt. Humans have no salt excretory glands, yet you have to get rid of the extra salt in sea water because the amount is just too much for your system. Your blood is not similar in composition to sea water (contrary to popular belief); your blood is several times more dilute. If your blood *were* like sea water, then you could safely drink sea water. In the process of excreting the excess salt in salt water, the human kidney draws water from the body's supply, a process so dehydrating that if sea water were the only fluid replacement available, you could die of thirst faster by drinking sea water than if you didn't. Human inability to drink sea water for fluid replacement is reflected in Samuel Taylor Coleridge's *Rime of the Ancient Mariner*—"Water, water everywhere, nor any drop to drink."

Preventing Dehydration

Your health benefits by good hydration. Bring plenty to drink on trips and hikes. Drink water throughout your day. Which drink you choose is a matter of personal taste. Try different drinks to determine which works best for you. Everyone's system differs in what it tolerates. Drink before you're thirsty. Sport drinks are quick and simple fluid, electrolyte, and carbohydrate replacement, and live up to claims for endurance events where you can't stop to eat or drink. For the general exerciser, they are not a magic energy food, but a good and easy way to keep hydrated.

17

Ergogenic Aids—Does Physical Enhancement Await on Your Plate?

Fillet of a fenny snake,
In the cauldron boil and bake;
Eye of newt and toe of frog,
Wool of bat and tongue of dog,
Adder's fork and blind-worm's sting,
Lizard's leg and owlet's wing,
For a charm of powerful trouble,
Like a hell-broth boil and bubble.

—Second Witch: *Macbeth,*
Act IV, Scene I

A miracle drug is any drug that will do what the label
says it will do.   —Eric Hodgins

The search for a personal edge that you can eat is a common one. Hundreds of years ago, Aztec warriors ate the hearts of fearless enemies, believing it would increase their own bravery. To prepare for battle, the Inca Indians chewed coca leaves, and Berserkers ate mushrooms containing muscarine. Norsemen drank the milk of Arctic reindeer in heat. In the Middle Ages, Dervishes whirled longer using coffee. Sigmund Freud used cocaine. Today, South American Indians know chewing coca leaves reduces hunger and fatigue. In the Middle East, khat leaves are chewed for similar effect, while in Asia and the South Pacific Islands it's betel nuts, and in the Sudan, the kola nut. Some people take diet pills, eat protein supplements, use steroids, drink coffee, or try preparations with labels promising everything from muscle growth to energetic hair.

What Is an Ergogenic Aid?

Products that help physical performance are called ergogenic aids. An *erg* is a unit of work. The word "energy" contains the erg root and means the ability to do work. The suffix *-gen* means "producing" or "generating." Putting them together forms the word "ergogenic" and refers to things used and, not incidentally, believed to enhance physical performance. Not everything claiming to be ergogenic is really ergogenic.

Some ergogenic aids are psychological, such as mental rehearsal, confidence training, and good-luck charms. Some are physical, such as swimming and lifting weights (don't forget that to get better physically, you can also work for it with exercise, not just by eating something). Nutritional ergogenic aids include an assortment of drugs, supplements, and food concoctions. The variety is ingenious, from broccoli pills to carbohydrate injections directly into muscle. Some are hokum—many products on the market claiming to be ergogenic have no ergogenic properties at all. Others work well enough to be banned by athletic associations and Olympic committees. A specific few present health hazards.

Why Do People Use Ergogenic Aids?

Would you pay to eat a product called "This Won't Work," or would you favor "Beautiful-Body-for-Certain"? Many people buy products sold through clever advertising and false hope. Product names are not required by law to do what they claim, allowing ads to combine suggestive words like *power, energy, natural, super,* and *mega* on their labels. Who could think a vitamin named Ener-B didn't have anything to do with feeling energetic? Ads targeting the serious bodybuilder market suggest anabolic steroid capability with names incorporating word segments like *ana, testo,* and *bolic.* Product promotions may include quotes from flawed studies in obscure or faux journals. The Food and Drug Administration (FDA) does not currently require testing these products for proof of efficacy. An athlete may work and slave, eat low fat, train diligently, but then attribute all gains to a capsule or pill, and go on to promote the product through testimonials.

Many stimulant preparations are sold as "natural" and "herbal." That does not mean they are harmless or nonaddictive. Cocaine and nicotine, for example, are naturally occurring plant substances. But many people buy stimulants thinking there will be no problems with them because they are labeled "natural."

"Natural" and "herbal" do not mean harmless or nonaddictive.

Another reason people use certain substances is that some of the potions work to various degrees. Some stimulants boost speed and endurance by increasing muscle contractility and/or energy use. Cardiac relaxants can improve aim in target shooting. Other substances increase muscle mass for strength and speed contests, increase endurance for long events, or just give an edge in the gym. Still others not only work, but are addictive like caffeine.

Stimulants

Stimulant drugs exert their effect directly on your nervous system. They are usually taken because they inhibit fatigue and appetite. Overstimulation and addiction are common, resulting in various effects that are not healthy.

Coffee

"Black as hell, strong as death, sweet as love," according to a Middle Eastern proverb. Few who drink tea, coffee, hot chocolate, or cola drinks consider themselves drug users. These drinks all contain caffeine, the most commonly used stimulant drug in the world. Other people shun caffeine, and instead take "natural" stimulant herbs (discussed below). Caffeine is no less "natural" than any health food herb. Caffeine was probably discovered in the Stone Age, and has been widely used ever since. Caffeine can extend endurance, and is banned in high concentrations by the International Olympic Committee for that reason. A big rage for caffeine as an ergogenic aid may have begun in 1978 when exercise physiologist David Costil, Ph.D., told *Runner's World* magazine that caffeine could improve marathon times. According to Professor of Medicine Randy Eichner, M.D., "This led to long coffee lines at big marathons, followed by long potty lines." How caffeine helps is still studied and debated. Caffeine is thought to help endurance by directly stimulating your central nervous system, decreasing your perception of effort, helping your body save some fuel called glycogen, and possibly, improving your use of fat as fuel. More recently, caffeine is thought to help short-term activity (so short that your body has no time to use either glycogen or fat) possibly by increasing recruitment of more of your muscle fibers and/or directly increasing their resistance to fatigue.

Some people react strongly to caffeine; others don't. That may be genetically based, and may change throughout your lifetime. It depends, of course, on dose, as well as metabolism, prior diet, fitness, and other interactions. For most people, nervousness, increased urine production, and heartbeat irregularities begin in the two- to three-cup range, with increasing tendency to irregular heart rhythms from caffeine as you get older. Side effects increase with dosage. Many preparations claiming energy effects from herbs contain caffeine or caffeine-like substances, so read labels carefully of any product claiming energy boosts.

If you don't already drink coffee or other caffeine drinks, there's no grounds to start just for an endurance boost. If you are a regular drinker, you may find the withdrawal symptoms of headache and weariness are not worth the effort to give it up for a day or week. Try to keep your use low to moderate, cut back if you comfortably can, and drink extra water to help offset the diuretic effect.

Sympathomimetic (sim-path-oh-my-MET-ik) Stimulants

Part of your nervous system increases heart rate and constricts blood vessels, getting you "ready to go." That part of your nervous system is called the sympathetic nervous system. Substances with properties that mimic your sympathetic nervous system are called sympathomimetic. Three examples are amphetamines, cocaine, and ma huang. (Caffeine and nicotine are not sympathomimetic. Not everything that is a central nervous system stimulant is sympathomimetic.)

Amphetamines More potent than coffee, amphetamines became popular as "pep pills" and diet pills because they mask tiredness and hunger. Amphetamines were given to soldiers during World War II to delay fatigue, and were widely used in medical practice until recently, when their dangers became widely known.

Amphetamine users may get abnormally high or irregular heart rates, raised blood pressure, and sometimes, mental states resembling paranoid schizophrenia. Abdominal cramps, incoordination, dizziness, dry mouth, nausea, and vomiting may also go along with initial use. Some people have unusual effects on their blood cells. Amphetamines constrict the arterioles of the skin (small, end branches of skin arteries), increasing risk of overheating. Deaths in endurance competitions in the heat have been connected to amphetamine use. Amphetamines usually physically and psychologically addict their user after about 12 weeks. Abusers can gradually increase their doses from 10 to 1,000 times to retain the initial effects they liked so much.

For weight control, diet pills are ineffective. They undermine sound nutrition and allow the user to ignore the requirement of exercise in fat reduction. Both the older amphetamine types and the newer diet pills require extreme caution and the care of a qualified physician. Moreover, after two to three weeks, diet pills begin losing effectiveness. Justifiable medical uses of amphetamines are treatment of narcolepsy and (arguably) attention deficit disorder in children. Packaged amphetamines come with a warning about decreased ability to do hazardous tasks like driving or operating machinery.

What's a good substitute for amphetamine drugs? Exercise. Exercise increases feelings of energy and offsets food calories for weight control.

Cocaine

Cocaine enhances physical performance, with an unhealthy price. Cocaine is sympathomimetic. Here's how it works: Your nerve endings release nerve transmission chemicals called catecholamines across a space, called a synapse, to the next nerve ending. After they have done their job to transmit their signal, you have to get the catecholamine back out of the synapse so it doesn't keep signaling and signaling. There are several normal mechanisms for that, including gathering the catecholamine back up into storage areas in the nerve endings, ready for more signaling at another time. Cocaine blocks this reuptake, prolonging the effects of released catecholamines. That's why you get so much signaling with cocaine. Lots of it. Signaling in some areas of your brain feels good.

As with other central nervous system stimulants, the extra signaling increases heart rate and muscle contraction, allowing more physical work, and making you feel "geared up" to do that work. Signaling to your heart and blood vessels, from the catecholamine called norepinephrine, raises blood pressure and increases abnormal heart beats. Too much of this can cause sudden heart attack, sometimes fatally.

Surviving that, the problem with not taking up your catecholamines again for reuse means that you can run out. Running out of your catecholamine stores leads to severe depression (the cocaine crash).

Many health foods and herbal remedies sold as "pick-me-ups" contain various central nervous system stimulants.

Ma Huang

Ma huang is an herb that has direct nervous system effects. It has been used medicinally in China for over 5,000 years. Many energy potions sold over the counter contain ma huang, for example *Diet Pep, Up Your Gas, Chi Power,* and *Jade Energy.* It comes from the ephedra plant, and contains ephedrine. You often find ephedrine in cold medications, to open airways and decrease secretions, and it is often used in treating allergies and asthma. Ma huang is sympathomimetic—it mimics activation of the sympathetic nervous system, mostly by releasing the catecholamines noradrenaline and adrenaline from nerve endings. As you might expect, overuse can lead to the serious side effects of raised heart rate and blood pressure.

Many people take ma huang as a pep pill, thinking it is somehow better or more "natural" than caffeine. But caffeine is as naturally occurring as ma huang, and both can have negative side effects in large dosages. Ma huang has recently come under scrutiny after causing several deaths from overstimulation of the heart. It should not be taken lightly.

Theobromine

Chocolate, gotu kola nut, and several other foodstuffs available in health food stores contain theobromine, among other substances. Theobromine stimulates the nervous system and increases heart rate, similar to caffeine, but less intensely. Theobromine is used in certain medicines and advertised in "health food" items promising "pep" for that reason.

Ginseng

Advertisements for herbal energy potions that say they are caffeine-free does not necessarily mean they are free of side effects or are healthy for you. Ginseng is an example. Because of ginseng's stimulant effects, it is popularly used for a variety of health problems, and for a general "pick-me-up." Ginseng is used in pills, teas, sodas, even candies. Ginseng can affect glucose metabolism, and raise heart rate and blood pressure. People who overmedicate themselves with ginseng can wind up with diarrhea, nervousness, skin rashes, and insomnia. Most of these symptoms will disappear when use is reduced or discontinued. This doesn't mean that ginseng is bad; just that it is not harmless. It has effects. That's why people take it.

Most of the biologic effects of ginseng come from the ginsenosides it contains. Investigations have found that content varies widely, with some ginseng preparations containing no ginsenosides at all. There is no law requiring uniformity, or even labeling to identify content.

Steroids and Steroid Substitutes

Anabolic Steroids

The word "anabolic" means that it promotes tissue growth. Not all steroids are anabolic. The antiinflammatories cortisone and prednisone are steroids and are not anabolic. They do not stimulate growth. Neither does Vitamin D, another steroid that is not an anabolic steroid.

Anabolic steroids are drugs that have anabolic and masculinizing or androgenic effects. Large muscle mass gains from oral and/or injectable forms don't routinely occur without intense strength training. Adverse physical and emotional side effects of anabolic steroids are common. Most are incompatible with physical and emotional health—high blood pressure, elevated "bad" cholesterol (LDL), liver and kidney damage, greater risk of heart and vascular disease, volatile aggressive "roid" rages, and reckless uncontrolled behaviors.

Growth Hormone

Growth hormone, abbreviated GH, has recently begun replacing steroids in popularity, probably because it is currently undetectable in drug tests. The American College of Sports Medicine (ACSM) strongly advises against GH for athletic enhancement because of ethical and physical problems.

GH in adults may irreversibly increase growth of the jaw, forehead, hands, and feet, even in cases where it has no effect to increase strength. It may also increase the risk of diabetes, high blood pressure, and heart problems.

Compounds supposedly having GH-releasing potential sell briskly in health food stores and gyms. Ornithine and Sapogenin are two growth hormone hopefuls that fall short. Ornithine is often packaged in 250 milligram capsules, although the effective dose is far higher. Sapogenins are derived from plants found in desert regions. Your body will excrete them without making any GH. If you want results similar to taking growth hormones, but in a natural, safe, and inexpensive manner without side effects, vigorous exercise does exactly that.

Anabolic Activators, Multipacs, and Enhancers

These are usually packs of food elements, labeled with the suggestive name "anabolic." They have no magical muscle-building abilities, and contain nothing that is not available in regular food. They are not steroid substitutes, except by name, and there is currently no law to prevent anyone from selling you potions called steroid substitutes, even if they have no anabolic steroid effect. The name "steroid substitute" only means that advertisers would like you to buy their products instead of steroids, not necessarily that the product works like them. The use of the word "anabolic" could technically mean that since some of these supplements have so many calories, they do promote tissue growth—of fat—the same way any other high-calorie food does. It's just snappy advertising.

Food Supplements

Protein

The most common belief about protein supplementation is that eating more protein will build you bigger muscles. It won't. Consider this. Protein enters into thousands of body functions besides muscle assembly. Eating more protein will not automatically increase all those functions. Protein builds skin, enters into the reactions that creates the pigment in your skin, and is a building block for the smooth muscle in your blood vessels. Extra protein doesn't grow you more skin, make you turn brown, or make your blood vessels more muscular.

Protein has many functions in your body besides growing
muscles. Eating more protein does not increase any of
those functions in speed or amount. For example, protein
is involved in pigmenting your skin, but eating more
protein does not darken your skin.

Do You Need More Protein When Active?

Studies find that for a brief time after beginning an exercise program, your body's protein balance falls, then restores to previous levels. Your need to increase protein (over the recommended minimum) may be brief and mild. Most people routinely eat more protein than the required recommended daily allowance (RDA). Because of all they already eat, any increased intake in meals or supplements is unnecessary.

You can't store protein the way you can store fat, and to a lesser extent, carbohydrate. Whenever you eat more protein than you need on any given day, most will convert to fat, and you will excrete the rest, a process requiring water. In high amounts, dietary protein contributes to dehydration.

For the average inactive person, the minimum RDA for protein is 0.8 grams for every kilogram of body weight. A kilogram is about 2.2 pounds, making your requirement less than half a gram of protein for every pound you weigh. The protein requirement for a 180-pound person (82 kilograms) person varies around 65 grams per day. That's only about 2 ounces. A 130-pounder (59 kilograms) meets minimum requirements with less than 50 grams.

An active athlete may need at least 1 gram per kilogram of body weight. Muscle magazines often state that you need a gram of protein or more per pound of body weight. This does not seem to be the case, and has not been shown to have any effect on muscle building. In fact, strength athletes usually need less protein than endurance athletes. It is the endurance athletes that need a bit more protein, as they burn more calories. Muscle requires little protein for growth. For active people, carbohydrate supplementation seems to be more important and contributes more to muscle building. *See* Chapter 14, "Nutrition Myths," for a closer look at protein.

Carbohydrates

Carbohydrates give you energy for all your activities. They are so important that your body stores them, mostly in your muscles and liver in a form called glycogen. The larger your stores, the longer you can exercise before you fatigue (depending on your physical fitness).

There are many energy bars, mixes, and drinks formulated to give you carbohydrates. They are not magic potions; they are food. Don't forget that you can also build and increase your normal carbohydrate stores when you regularly exercise and eat regular meals of at least 60% carbohydrate.

Because athletes exercising at high intensities for long periods can delay fatigue and therefore work longer and harder with carbohydrates, including carbohydrate drinks, misunderstandings result. Taking carbohydrate drinks and preparations will not transform you into a better athlete. Your ability to do submaximal exercise like recreational running, swimming, biking, dancing, walking, skating, and so on, does not improve from any particular food or drink.

Carbohydrate Loader Drinks. Carbohydrate loader drinks are one of several kinds of sport drinks. Carbohydrate loader drinks have a higher carbohydrate content than regular electrolyte replacer drinks. Loader drinks have three main applications:

1. During intense, long-duration exercise they provide fuel to delay fatigue.
2. For athletes who work out so much that they can't maintain their weight with regular meals and snacks, the drinks add calories.
3. For people unable to eat a regular meal before physical activity because of time restraints or jittery stomach, the drinks become a temporary meal substitute or adjunct.

Carbohydrate loader drinks are not magic energy elixirs or stimulants. They won't give you a performance edge if taken before or during exercise much shorter than an hour or so, like an aerobics class, a half hour to hour of cycling, skiing, or basketball, or even a 6–10-kilometer jog. Athletes generally have enough of their own stored carbohydrate, called glycogen, to last about an hour to 90 minutes. Carbohydrate drinks are most effective to delay fatigue when carbohydrate concentration is between 6% and 8% and when exercise is tough stuff lasting over an hour. The commercial drink Bodyfuel 450®, for example, is 4.5% carbohydrate, Gatorade® is 6.0%, and Exceed® is 7.0%.

Carbohydrate Replacer Drinks. Carbohydrate replacement drinks are another kind of sport drink useful for replacing carbohydrates after exercise. They have a higher carbohydrate content than the loader drinks. Long, intense exercise depletes glycogen, an important fuel. Replacement drinks help restock your muscle and liver glycogen after hard activity. You need to replace glycogen as soon as possible after exercise. If you don't, your body can't make enough glycogen to replace the loss. Your muscle and liver reserves remain low even days later, limiting further exercise ability.

The first 30 minutes after hard exercise are crucial to the major restocking. Your muscles can restore more total carbohydrate if you begin to eat or drink carbohydrates within 30 minutes after hard exercise. The next two hours are the second important stage. You benefit by eating high-carbohydrate food as soon after exercise as you can. Unfortunately, many people get changed, pack away their gear, and return home before eating anything. By then a critical maximum restock window has passed. For this reason, high-carbohydrate replacement drinks were developed for right after exercise. Eating your ordinary meals and drinking extra water would do just as well. Replacement drinks serve the market for those who prefer to drink rather than eat right after exercise, or who just want something prepackaged and ready to swallow. Sport drinks make a handy after-exercise snack. Their high carbohydrate content means the drinks are high calorie. Don't go overboard with these, or the extra calories will store not as glycogen, but fat.

Bee Pollen

Bee pollen is claimed to have all sorts of effects, from vague "vitality" to specific athletic improvements. Bee pollen has not been experimentally shown to enhance any aspect of athletic performance or have any effect on your level of physical stimulation. It does cause allergic reactions in susceptible people, and has caused some deaths.

Enyzmes

Enzymes are large protein molecules. Your body manufactures many hundreds of enzymes that are involved in every reaction in your body. Does that mean that you can buy a bottle of enzymes to increase specific reactions in your body? For example, there are enzymes that increase oxygen use during exercise. There are other enzymes that reduce the harmful free radicals that are accepted to cause many problems. Can eating more of these enzymes increase your athletic ability or decrease your risk of these problems? No.

If you eat bottled enzymes, your digestive system will break them apart into their component proteins to make them small enough to pass though your small intestine into your bloodstream. The breaking-down process destroys them as enzymes. Component protein molecules are not automatically reassembled into enzymes on the other side of the intestinal wall.

It's useless to eat bottled enzymes—and expensive. Important exceptions are those enzymes that work before passing through the intestine, used to aid digestion. One example is Lactaid, the enzyme that breaks down lactose in milk, and so, prevents the gas and bloating common in adults who no longer digest dairy products well. *See* Chapter 14, "Nutrition Myths," for more about antioxidants and oxygen toxicity.

Taking enzyme pills for energy or other health claims is completely useless.
Your digestive system breaks enzymes apart before they get into your bloodstream. They are no longer enzymes, and will not reassemble into enzymes.

Vitamins

Many people regard vitamins as ergogenic aids. No scientific evidence supports vitamin supplementation as ergogenic. Unless you have a nutritional deficiency, increasing your intake will not improve your physical abilities. There are plenty of important roles for vitamins, but study after study demonstrates that ergogenics is not one of them.

Vitamins have no calories, so furnish no energy, by definition. Vitamins are often advertised as giving energy, even labeled with suggestive names like "Ener-B." Unless your fatigue relates to a deficiency, they will not make you energetic.

Vitamin B_{12} has been called the least likely vitamin to affect
sport performance and the most likely to be abused for
nonexistent ergogenic effects.

Taking too many vitamins can be unhealthy. Some vitamins are fat-
soluble. With repeated overdosing they can accumulate in your body
to toxic levels. Other vitamins are water-soluble and you excrete them,
but can still have side effects with long-term overdose.

Minerals

Like vitamins, minerals have no calories and no known ergogenic
effects. Deficiencies may result in weaknesses, but taking amounts
above your needs will not improve your physical fitness. Even so,
many have been advertised with claims of ergogenic effects.

Boron is one of several minerals misrepresented as an ergogenic
aid. A widely misquoted study found low dietary boron decreased
testosterone in postmenopausal women. Levels rose when the deficiency was corrected. From that came many claims of boron as helpful
to athletes to increase their testosterone levels, with "studies" seeming
to back up those claims. Although problems stem from nutrient deficiency, there is no evidence that extra boron elevates testosterone.
Large doses are toxic. Boron is an ultratrace mineral. You need only
tiny amounts, and can get it from fruits, vegetables, nuts, and legumes.

Chromium (including chromium picolinate) and vanadium are also
ultratrace minerals in the diet. If a deficiency exists, the benefit of
supplementation is to correct the deficiency. There's no good evidence
that they otherwise alter your body composition, or enhance athletic
ability to any extent that it matters to most exercisers.

Carnitine

The excitement over carnitine began when the Italian soccer team
won a title while taking carnitine. Obviously, the team did many other
things beside taking carnitine, like train at high levels. There was no
real evidence to show the carnitine had anything to do with their
season outcome, yet such advertising sells many bottles of carnitine.

Your body makes its own carnitine, and distributes it to many of your body's cells. Primarily it works to carry unoxidized fatty acids. There is a D form and an L form. Those initials just tell how the molecule rotates—to the right (dextro-, or D-rotatory) or left (levo-rotatory, or L form). Eating too much of the D form of carnitine in supplements can make you lose the L form. In this case, supplementation can be harmful.

It's difficult to become deficient in carnitine through training. There's no good evidence that taking carnitine, in any of its forms, does much that can be considered very helpful, but there is also not enough evidence to reject it completely. Some studies do show very small gains. For the small gains and big price tag, the average exerciser can get just as much gain through regular exercise.

Carbohydrate Injection

Korean speed skaters are reported to have been experimenting with glycogen injections directly into thigh muscle. The unanswered question for elite athletes is can it do any good? The answer for regular exercisers is that it is completely unnecessary in any case.

Fluid Retention

Fluid retention has been examined as an ergogenic aid. The theory is that muscle leverage favorably changes as the muscle swells with extra water. You can increase your total body water in several ways—carbohydrate loading increases the water your muscles can hold, eating salt retains more water, and anabolic steroids swell you with water, before they have a chance to exert any androgenic effect.

But should you count on fluid retention to help you in sports or exercise? Most people don't drink enough water, which is a common, and hidden, cause of fatigue. Getting enough water is a good idea and can make you feel better by itself. As far as dosing on extra water, the effect would be small, if any. Your body will usually regulate things so that any excess is quickly eliminated.

Water

The most overlooked athletic ability aid is water. You need to replace body water before and after activity, and during long activities, particularly in the heat. Water is a good, inexpensive, and easy fluid replacer for exercise, and for daily activities. Try to drink eight glasses of water every day, more when exercising in the heat. Drinking good, clean water is healthy, and can even help control your appetite.

What Will Give You an Advantage?

Overwhelming evidence points to regular good nutrition, good hydration, and regular exercise, not supplements for athletic advantage. What can you do?

- Trade high-protein, high-fat, low-carbohydrate burgers for moderate-protein, low-fat, high-complex-carbohydrate meals whenever you can.
- Get enough protein. Don't eat only a salad for lunch or coffee and Danish for breakfast. Get protein throughout the day, rather than only at dinner.
- Eat frequent, healthy meals. Don't starve yourself.
- Eat breakfast.
- Rest is a greatly ignored ergogenic aid. Get your R&R—get enough sleep and enjoy your life.
- Exercise for fun and health.
- Drink water.
- Add up all the money you save on supplements.
- Be good to yourself—possibly the most neglected of personal enhancing devices.

18

Healthy Eating

A food is not necessarily essential just because your child hates it.

—Katherine Whitehorn

Eating nutrition-poor food is common. Sometimes unhealthy foods are the only offerings at restaurants, movies, ball games, theme parks, and public events. Unhealthy eating is so easy to do and so well accepted as normal that it often goes unnoticed as a major factor in fatigue, extra pounds, and some of the most common Western diseases including cardiovascular disease, diverticulitis, and diabetes. Many people turn to vitamins and health food products hoping these will fix their low energy or poor health, without ever looking at unhealthy daily eating habits behind their problem.

This chapter looks at a few common eating habits that lead to weight gain, fatigue, and health problems. It explains what to do about it, some myths of healthy and unhealthy eating, and how simple, good-tasting choices can improve your health.

Eating Backwards in Quantity

Eating backwards is a common bad nutrition habit. People often eat backwards two main ways. The first is quantity.

Healthy eaters have larger breakfasts and lunches, and smaller dinners. People who eat backward in quantity do the opposite—they eat little or nothing for breakfast, rush off to work, have little for lunch, take candy and coffee breaks during the day, then eat a large supper at night and a snack or two later on. The result is often fatigue during and after work, candy cravings, crankiness, and extra pounds.

You may feel fatigued when you don't eat enough food at the beginning and middle of the day. You need carbohydrate energy to work, do physical activity, and get around enough to enjoy life. Although many people hope their bodies will burn fat if they cut back breakfast, your body first turns to its protein stores, not fat, when dietary carbohydrate is low. Low-carbohydrate breakfasts and lunches often lead to snacks of candy. Sugary snacks are high calorie, and may contribute to mood swings in those people susceptible to low blood sugar–induced crankiness. Large high-protein and high-fat meals at night add more calories, protein, and fat when you need less.

Eating Backwards in Quality

The second main way people eat backwards concerns what they eat. Sometimes people have good-sized breakfasts, but filled with fat. They may stuff themselves on eggs, sausage, bacon, and pastry. Backwards meals are 40–50% fat, up to 30% and more of protein, but little of an important nutrient—complex carbohydrate. Eating backwards in quality, as with quantity, often results in fatigue. You haven't supplied your body with enough complex carbohydrates for energy. Nutrition surveys find that many people eat backwards in quality. Healthy meals have most of the calories, about 50–60%, as complex carbohydrate, less than 30% fat, and the rest protein, depending on your body weight.

Typical Backwards Meals

A typical day of backwards meals begins with no breakfast, or a breakfast of coffee or tea, pastry or donuts, or eggs and sausage. Then a sugary snack at a midmorning coffee break because of low energy. Lunch may be a burger and fries—high fat and high protein, but low complex carbohydrate. Another late afternoon sugary/fatty donut or cookie snack because you are starving for sugar, a large high-protein, high-fat dinner with high-fat ice cream, cake, or pie for dessert, and often a sugary snack (or two) of cookies and maybe some potato chips later that night to calm rebounding low blood sugar from earlier candy snacks.

Why Do People Eat Backwards?

Why do people eat backwards this way? A big reason, unfortunately, is the U.S. Department of Agriculture's old four food groups, two of which are the high-fat meat and dairy groups. There is good evidence that humans did not evolve eating high amounts of meat. Dairy is also a relatively late evolutionary addition to the adult diet. Modern, Western diets often have meat and dairy every day, sometimes every meal. The human body is not designed to handle it all. Meat is not only protein, as often thought. Bacon, for example, can have around 80% of its calories as fat. Many meats are over 50% fat. (*See* Chapter 15, "Calculating Food Fat.")

On April 9, 1991, the Physicians' Committee for Responsible Medicine released a statement that a diet based on the old four food groups will not ensure adequate nutrition, and promotes disease. This is not new information. A 1978 study showed that only 9 of 17 minimum daily required amounts of needed nutrients were met by meals based on the old four food groups. The 1977–78 Nationwide Food Consumption Survey stated, "Americans who eat diets based on the four food groups consume an excessive amount of fat."

Another reason for backwards eating habits is that many people still remember when complex carbohydrates used to be called starches. They regard complex carbohydrate as fattening food to avoid.

A third reason is that often the only food available at restaurants, office buildings, ballparks, picnics, and drive-throughs is nutritionally backwards packaged foods and popular fast foods, all high fat and low carbohydrate.

Yet another reason is habit. The most popular snack foods of packaged chips and lunch meats are backwards, but become habits at early ages. People eat these because they are part of their daily routines.

Food preparation can add fat to previously not-so-bad foods, for example, adding sour cream, butter, and cheese to a baked potato.

Then there are honest mistakes. Food is often labeled as health food to make it sell, when it is high fat, such as granola bars.

Is It Natural?

Eating high fat is a common bad nutrition habit. It is easy to do, and becomes natural. The taste perception of people accustomed to fat changes to the point where food that isn't fatty doesn't taste as good to them. People who switch from whole-fat milk to non-or low-fat milk say that the lower-fat product tastes watery at first. After an adjustment period, the same people tasting whole-fat milk again often protest that the high-fat item tastes too fatty, like drinking butter, which is not all that far from truth. Whole milk, though labeled 3% fat, is in truth, close to 50% fat by calories. (*See* Chapter 15, "Calculating Food Fat.")

Children fed high-fat and highly sugared foods develop the habit of eating them. When visiting anthropologists gave South American Indian children candy, the children spit it out as bad tasting. Although our bodies have an evolutionary survival tendency to prefer sugar and fat foods, foods as high in fat and sugar as we now eat didn't exist until recently. Many modern food preferences are often just habit.

How to Make Bad Food Habits into Good Ones

Eating healthy should not be some hateful thing you do at certain meals because you have to, then discard the rest of the time to go back to your "real" foods. Like exercise, healthy eating can gradually become a good-tasting, normal way of life. Good eating habits are something that you can make a part of ordinary daily living.

Don't Eat Backwards

Healthy eaters have larger breakfasts and lunches, and smaller dinners. Healthy meals have most of the calories, about 60%, as complex carbohydrate, have less than 30% fat, and about 12–16% protein, depending on your body weight.

New Food Groups

Recently, the old four food groups were replaced by a seven-group food pyramid. Smaller groups include a sugar and fat group to be eaten sparingly, and a protein group that includes beans and meat.

Large helpings of fruits, grains, and vegetables form the large, solid base of the pyramid. The new recommendations agree on vegetables as main dishes, with meat as side dishes if you eat meat. Not the other way around.

Figure 18.1. The new food pyramid replaces the old four food groups. The new food pyramid emphasizes less fat, shown by putting it at the small end of the pyramid. More main meals of vegetables, fruits, grains, and legumes (foods like beans, lentils, and peas) form the large, supporting base.

Serving Sizes

Eating good food is one of life's great pleasures. Getting into shape and losing weight does not mean giving up that pleasure. It means learning a little portion control.

Eating is one of life's pleasures. With regular exercise and rational portions, you can have your cake and eat it, too.

The food pyramid talks about "serving size" but what is that? In theory it is one thing, but in practice, people eat far more than they think.

	Official USDA Serving	Typical Restaurant Serving
Ice cream	½ cup	1 cup+
Meat	3 oz	6–16 oz
Salad dressing	2 tbsp	4 tbsp
Slice of pizza	5 oz	9 oz+
Muffin	2 oz	4–6 oz
French fries	3 oz	6–8 oz+

Eat Breakfast

A healthy habit is to eat breakfasts of high complex carbohydrate, some fat, and moderate protein to fuel the day's work and exercise.

Eat Snacks

Animals like snakes and lions go long periods between meals. Humans seem to be natural snackers. Done right, snacking can help keep weight and food cravings down, and energy up. Frequent, low-volume eating is sometimes called grazing. The human body may have evolved to favor grazing between meals. If done with healthy foods, the body seems to adjust to more total calories without as much weight gain compared to eating the same number of calories in one or two daily meals. Two important things happen, among many, when time interval increases between meals. In the short term, blood sugar goes down, signaling hunger. In the long term, your body learns it must hold tightly to the fat it gets to survive. When meals are frequent, the body learns there will always be more coming down the tube. There is less survival-based need to hold on to each incoming calorie.

Try snacks like fruit, bagels, vegetables, pretzels, breads, and air-popped popcorn during the day for energy. Make complex carbohydrates the majority of your calories, about 60%, in your regular meals.

Eating Before Activity

Some people can eat just about anything before exercising. Others can't stomach meals before activity, particularly not before strenuous activity. If you don't tolerate a regular meal before exercise, try small snacks of bagels, fruit, sport bars, raisins, hard pretzels, and commercially available liquid meals and sport drinks. Experiment to find a balance that is right for you.

Choosing What to Eat

Protein

The amount of protein you need depends on your body weight. Most people in the Western nations get more protein than they need. Any extra protein you eat does not automatically convert into muscle. Extra protein also will not build you bigger muscles with exercise than if you didn't eat extra protein. If you stop exercising, eating extra protein will not make you keep the muscles you have. Without exercise, your muscles will shrink in size but they do not turn into fat. Muscle cells still stay muscle cells, just smaller ones.

Grains and vegetables are just fine as protein sources. You don't have to carefully mix them to get the right proportions of proteins, as once thought.

As a minimum, eat about 0.8 to 1.0 grams of protein for every kilogram you weigh. If you weigh 130 pounds (59 kg), get at least 47 grams of protein every day. If you weigh 150 pounds (68 kg), get at least 54 grams of protein. If you weigh 170 pounds (77 kg), get a minimum of 61 grams. If you weigh 200 pounds (90 kg), get 73 grams of protein.

You can find the gram content of protein on the food labels. You do not need much more protein with heavy exercise, but you do need more carbohydrate in order to fuel that exercise. Find out more about protein and protein myths in Chapter 14, "Nutrition Myths."

Fat

The American Heart Association calls for keeping fat under 20–30% at most, with most of that nonsaturated vegetable fat. High blood fats are thought to impede circulation. Chronically narrowed blood vessels from high-fat diets are no help to you either. Extremely low-fat diets, those of about 10% fat, have been found not only to stop advancing heart disease, but to help reverse it. You don't need to cut out fat entirely. A little fat is important to healthy eating.

Complex Carbohydrates

They used to be called starches. It's a myth that starch is fattening. Too many calories from any source is fattening, but complex carbohydrates are healthy eating and, like fiber, found only in plants. Make them around 60% or so of your calories, more before strenuous activities. Eat more baked, boiled, and steamed potatoes, rice, beans, broccoli, bread, fruit, grain cereals, pasta, salads, and whole grains.

Can Carbs Make You Fat?

What about the recent "carbo-bashing" starting with a *New York Times* article, "Eating Pasta Makes You Fat," and the wide media coverage that followed? The concern was that emphasizing carbohydrates would exacerbate "Syndrome X" in "insulin-resistant" people, an estimated 10–25% of Americans.

"Syndrome X" is a collection of risk factors for heart disease including high blood pressure, low "good cholesterol," high triglycerides, and obesity. "Insulin resistance" is a topic with a lot of unknowns in it. It seems to involve a reduced number of insulin receptors. Body cells don't know how much insulin they already got delivered. The pancreas secretes more and more insulin, not knowing when to stop. In theory, this insulin oversecretion causes the carbohydrates to be better stored as fat.

At the heart of the public's confusion were missing facts:

- Carbohydrate will only store as fat if you eat too much of it.
- Even "insulin-resistant" people must eat excess carbohydrate calories before the carbohydrates are stored as fat.
- Losing excess weight and increasing physical activity are far more important in controlling insulin resistance than restricting carbohydrates.
- In most cases, insulin resistance seems to be caused by excess weight and inactivity, not the other way around.

What about the now-famous attack on pasta when fetuccine Alfredo was named "heart attack on a plate"? That was the high-fat, artery-clogging sauce. Other pasta dishes suffered guilt by association.

Fiber

Fiber used to be called roughage. Fiber is the most complex of complex carbohydrates. So complex that your digestive system can't digest it. That's why fiber passes through your system, with healthy effects on your lower intestinal tract. Fiber is found only in plants, not in meat, poultry, fish, eggs, or dairy. Get lots of water-soluble fiber in oats, fruit, barley, and beans. Get insoluble fiber in vegetables and wheat.

Simple Sugars

Save for special occasions, not daily use. You'll be surprised that you crave them less as you consume less.

Handy Tips

If you are a beef and ale kind of eater, you don't want to be told to give that all up and eat carrots. You won't do it anyway. The good news is you don't have to. Some simple easy suggestions follow for making healthy eating a regular habit, not a hateful, tasteless thing you do because it's good for you. You don't have to choose between being happy and being healthy. Have both. Make them the same thing.

From the following suggestions, choose a few things to start with for new healthy eating habits. Then add others as you can and want.

- Eat breakfast.
- Tea and toast, or coffee and Danish for breakfast won't fuel you and can leave you irritable and craving sugar hours later. Eat complex carbohydrates and protein for breakfast. Good examples are oatmeal, pancakes, hot and cold grain cereals, and fresh fruit.
- Try eating larger meals in the morning and afternoon, and smaller meals in evening. Most people eat backwards, eating little during the day and much at night.
- Keep healthy snacks handy like fruit, bagels, small amounts of raisins and almonds mixed together, breads, grains, pastas, hard pretzels, and others.
- Learn about the new food pyramid.
- Avoid fad diets that omit major food categories. They are nutritionally unsound and don't work in the long run. You don't lose fat that way, but you will lose water, muscle, bone, and other things you need.
- Get an air popcorn popper.

- Eat lightly before exercise—don't go hungry. Experiment to find foods and time schedules that agree with you if you have a tender tummy.
- Drink water with every meal. Drink extra water when exercising, particularly exercising in the heat.
- Have vegetables as main dishes with meat as side dishes, not the other way around.
- Make your involvement with healthy eating a stress-free one. It makes no sense for your body and mind to be miserable in the name of health. Take a happy approach. Make sure your new program is one that suits you.
- Use seasonings rather than butter or sour cream dressings. Use nonstick sprays instead of thick layers of butter and oil in the pan.
- If you make your own juice, keep the fruit pulp in the juice, rather than throwing it out. The complex carbohydrates, vitamins, and fiber in the pulp are healthy eating and help keep blood sugar stable. Without the fruit pulp, juices are little more than flavored sugar water.
- Find healthy foods you love. Don't be miserable with your new plan to eat right. Find ways that make your stomach happy as well as your conscience.
- Good-tasting, healthier recipes are available for old favorite, but unhealthy foods. Take a walk to the bookstore for a few fun books.
- Be good to yourself—possibly the most neglected healthy habit.

A Major Part of Healthy Living

Make healthy eating an enjoyable lifestyle, not just something to try for a day then stop because you've done it (and you hate it). Of course, there's more to health and energy than only eating right. It helps to inherit some healthy genes, to surround yourself with favorable environmental factors like exercise, clean water, air, and happiness, and to avoid smoking, nonmedicinal drugs, and too much alcohol. But remember that healthy eating is a major foundation of good health. Summing it up, that's nature, nurture, and nutrition. Or genes, means, and beans.

19

How to Lose Weight Without Dieting

Eat less than you think you want, eat with your intelligence, not your stomach. Never get up from the table with an inward, silent apology for being a pig.

—Coco Chanel

Never eat more than you can lift.

—Miss Piggy

Having a little extra body fat is helpful for warmth, cushioning, and buoyancy in the water. Losing extra weight can benefit your joints, cardiovascular system, and your general health and well-being. Sometimes it is even crucial. But severe calorie restriction and fad diets can be unhealthy, and they rarely work to maintain weight loss on a long-term basis.

There is no need to choose between the problems of being too heavy and the misery of dieting. You can do many things to lose weight without starving yourself or eating foods you hate. Good exercise and nutrition habits can become an easy, fun part of your lifestyle with attention and repetition.

Don't go at it without a plan. Aimlessly trying "diets" or vowing to "lose weight" does not work. It's not enough to say, "I'll lose ten pounds by next month." You need definite goals, methods to carry them out, and a schedule. Most important, you first need to take a good hard look at the way you eat now, and how much activity you get.

Cut Back Fats

Reducing fat in your diet can help you lose weight. Eating less saturated fat also may reduce your risk of heart disease and some cancers.

According to some studies, cutting back fat is a better way to lose weight than just cutting calories. Some of the reasoning for this idea is that your body uses fewer calories to digest fat than it does to digest carbohydrate. High-fat meals end up as fat on your body more readily than high-carbohydrate meals with the same number of calories. The human body is designed to store fat, and more easily stores it when provided directly. That doesn't mean you can eat high-calorie meals every day as long as they are low fat. The extra calories will just turn into fat in your body.

Many of your food choices may be high fat without you knowing it, like muffins and granola bars. Other foods that you know are high fat may be higher than you realized, like bacon, which can be around 80% fat. *See* Chapter 15, "Calculating Food Fat," to find out just how much fat many popular foods have. Take a good, hard look at what you eat, and where all the extra calories are coming from.

Substitute

Don't deny yourself food—substitute a lower-calorie for a higher-calorie food. When you are about to eat foods full of sugar and fat, eat something lower calorie instead—grains, fruits, and vegetables. Complex carbohydrates used to be called starches and were avoided. We now understand that eating sensible amounts of complex carbohydrates, rather than too much fat and sugar, is a key to healthier eating. Be creative and find things you like.

- Try substituting pretzels instead of potato chips, raisins instead of candy, bananas instead of banana cake, rolls instead of donuts.
- Fry less; bake, boil, and steam more.
- Use nonstick spray instead of butter, margarine, or oil.
- If you must use oil, use less than usual, and choose unsaturated oils like olive oil, instead of butter.
- If you have to have butter, choose whipped butter—it has more air and a bit fewer calories, or try "light" butter. Or use seasonings instead of butter.

- Instead of pouring oil on your salad, try balsamic vinegar, pureed cucumbers, seasonings, and low-fat yogurt, or even hot sauce.
- Try steam-sautéing in soup stock.
- Instead of cream on your potato, try lemon pepper seasoning, soy sauce, or nonfat sour cream.
- Strain plain yogurt to make a creamy, cream cheese substitute.
- You can buy nonfat sour cream and nonfat ice cream as easily as high-fat brands.
- For sweet desserts, try fruit and frozen yogurt, instead of pie and ice cream.
- Get applesauce without added sugar or syrup. It is plenty sweet. Add cinnamon. Or nutmeg. Use over oatmeal instead of sugar, and over fruit for dessert and snacks.
- Try chili powder and other seasonings, including low-calorie butter-flavored seasonings, instead of butter on air-popped popcorn.
- Use aromatic foods to flavor sauces instead of butter, cream, or cheese. Such aromatic flavorful foods include tomatoes, onions, garlic, mushrooms, leeks, fresh parsley, thyme, and basil.
- Many favorite recipes, particularly baked goods, use large amounts of fat to retain moisture during cooking. When you bake, substitute fruit such as applesauce, bananas, or prunes for most of the oil and sugar. These fruits will make your baking sweet and moist with much less fat and sugar.
- Instead of high-fat dairy, substitute mashed tofu, which is high-protein, high-calcium, and has no cholesterol.
- Refrigerate soups and stocks to separate and congeal the fat, skim it off, and use the skimmed product instead.
- Make yolkless omelets. A three egg-white omelet, prepared with nonstick spray and seasonings, has about 50 calories and no fat. A three-egg omelet has 225 calories and 15 grams of fat.
- Make baked apple with cinnamon instead of sugar or honey. It will be plenty sweet.
- If all else fails, and you know you are eating when you are not hungry, drink a large glass of water, then brush your teeth instead of snacking. The water will fill your stomach, and few people will eat with the fresh taste of toothpaste in their mouth.

Don't Go Hungry

Fasting and semistarvation diets make your body hang on to its fat stores. They also make you hungry and unhappy. Starving yourself, then snitching candy, can make you moody and craving to eat everything you see, usually in the late afternoons, then again at night.

Don't skip meals. Eat low-fat, sensible complex carbohydrate snacks in midmorning and late afternoon. Eat complex carbohydrates often to help maintain steady blood sugar levels. Don't just eat "low-fat" cakes. They are full of simple sugar, which will make you hungry within a few hours.

Less Simple Sugar

Eat complex carbohydrates like fruit and bagels for snacks instead of candy, and high-protein, high-complex-carbohydrate oatmeal instead of donuts and Danish for breakfast. When you eat less sugar, a magic thing happens—you crave less. Keep a list if you have to, to see what you eat every day. Find out where all the extra sugar you eat is coming from.

Be Prepared

You may have created a healthy cupboard and refrigerator for yourself at home, but most offerings away from home at fast-food places, restaurants, the workplace, public events, and snack machines are high fat, high sugar, and low complex carbohydrate. Go prepared. Pack fruit and bagels to snack, so you don't wind up with fries, shakes, and candy. Or pack a pasta lunch (cooked without oil or cream sauces), lentils, or other grains, with seasonings rather than oil. Other options are the many commercial sport nutrition bars and drinks. Some are no more than candy with a sporty name; others are genuine, good, healthy food.

Sport bars and drinks are not magic energy potions; they are just regular food in a wrapper. Read labels critically to find those that are low fat. They usually come in at least a few flavors, are easy to throw in a briefcase or bag, and make a quick, easy snack, a small meal in emergencies, or meal adjunct.

Make It Easy

It's easier to reach into the refrigerator or cupboard and pull out a cookie or cake than take the time to fix a healthy meal. Have healthy food ready and easy to get to. Keep a bowl of fruit handy. Make healthy snacks ahead of time for when you know you will eat impulsively, and put them on the top shelf of the refrigerator, and in the front of your cupboards.

Take Your Time

Lose weight the way you gained it—slowly. It will pay. Think long term. Food items are not worked off in single death-bouts. Don't get discouraged if your body is not remade by the end of a week, or a month. Small daily calorie expenditures multiply over time. An easy 150-calorie-a-day walk translates into about 15 pounds a year. Remember that it works both ways—one extra 150-calorie-a-day piece of candy can mean you weigh 15 pounds more in one year. Make that work for you with slow, steady reduction that does not tax your system. Slow weight loss is more likely to stay off, is easier on your heart, and spares bone and muscle.

Check for Extra Calories You Don't Need

You can cut many calories by not tasting foods as much when you cook, not licking icing from spoons, or "just" breaking off halves of cookies to snack on throughout the day. It can add up to hundreds of calories each day. Sometimes all it takes to lose the 10 or 20 pounds you want is to cut out one regular bedtime snack. Stopping one 300–400-calorie-a-night snack will make a quite a difference. Try not to eat close to bedtime.

Remember That "Diet Food" Is Food

Foods labeled as "diet food" are not magic potions that remove fat and calories from your body. They do not make you thinner just by the action of eating them. They are food. Regular food. They have calories. They can make you fat if you eat too much of them.

More Physical Activity

The major factor in overweight is a sedentary lifestyle. If you reduce your activity enough to gain only one pound per year, think how much heavier you will be in 20 years. Now think about only two pounds per year. These are pounds you will probably not notice on a day-to-day basis. Small things add up. Responsible plans for long-term weight loss include exercise. Exercise, in almost all cases, is a healthier, more effective weight loss method than starving yourself. A University of California study found that most of those able to remain slimmed down were those who started exercising regularly.

Figure 19.1. The major cause of overweight is inactivity.

Some people prefer organized exercise classes. They will drive to go to a gym and take the elevator to an exercise class, but hate to go out for a walk. Others haven't access or time to go to a gym, or they just hate the idea. Fortunately for them, getting in shape doesn't automatically mean three punishing sieges per week, pulse checks, group humiliation, and regimentation. Find an activity you like anyway, like going to a dance club, bicycling, or walking. Then you don't have to go to a gym just to get activity. Make your life active. Try all kinds of things until you find something you love to do.

The modern inactive life goes against the evolutionary
history and design of the human body to be active.
Going to a gym today is only a substitute for a natural
active life.

Want to burn more calories, even at work? The day is loaded with opportunities. If you drive to work, park farther away and walk the rest. Why wait for an elevator when you can improve your legs on the stairs? You may beat the elevator. If you work on an upper floor, take the elevator a few flights and walk the rest. Hand-deliver interoffice mail any chance you have. Instead of a smoke break, or donut and Danish break, take a walk and stretch break. Even people so heavy that any activity is difficult can find something that they can do. *See* Chapter 13, "How to Get Started Getting In Shape," and Chapter 26, "What to Do About the Shape You're In," for more on exercise ideas for weight control.

When you think about it, the human body was designed for activity, and was active through the eons. Modern life became inactive, bringing diseases of inactivity with it. Going to the gym is just a substitute for having an activity level that seems to be programmed into the human body for health. With some practice, you can find activities that are fun, and do them often, until they become a natural, healthy aspect of your life.

Being more active is the key to weight control. Find ways to be more active as part of your everyday life.

Make It Fun

All the ways listed above to control your weight without diets can become easy, safe, good-tasting, even fun, lifetime habits that work. Eat healthy and increase your daily activity level by making common lifetime activities part of your exercise. It will pay off in a lifetime of enjoyment.

How to Lose Weight Without Killing Yourself

Cut Back Fats. There are obvious ways you get too much fat, like fried food, rich desserts, and using full-fat dairy products, and there are ways you don't realize—creams and oils in sauces, salads, and snacks.

Substitute. Substitute good-tasting healthy foods for unhealthy ones. Be creative and find foods you like.

Don't Go Hungry. Starving yourself makes you hungry and unhappy, and makes your body hang on to its fat stores.

Don't Skip Meals. Eat healthy snacks, not candy or cakes, to help maintain steady blood sugar levels.

Less Simple Sugar. When you eat less sugar, you crave less.

Be Prepared. Pack healthy food to take with you to places that have only unhealthy food.

Make It Easy. Have healthy food ready and easier to get to than junk food when you know you will eat impulsively.

Take Your Time. Slow weight loss is more likely to stay off, is easier on your heart, and spares bone and muscle.

Check for Extra Calories You Don't Need. Sometimes all it takes to lose the 10 or 20 pounds you want is to cut out idle snacking.

Remember That "Diet Foods" Are Food. They do not make you thinner just by eating them. They can make you fat if you eat too much of them.

More Physical Activity. The major factor in overweight is a sedentary lifestyle.

Make It Fun. Make your new healthy lifestyle a fun one so that you stay with it, and enjoy it.

Resources for Low-Fat Cooking

There are many low-fat cookbooks. One very good, quick, and easy one is:

Low on the Go—Quick, Low Fat Recipes for Busy People
By Terri Peterson
$15.95 plus $3 postage (MD residents add 5% tax)
Lean for Life
P.O. Box 264
Olney, MD 20830-0264

Part Three

Health

A person ought to handle his body like the sail of a ship, and neither lower and reduce it much when no cloud is in sight, nor be slack and careless in managing it when he comes to suspect something is wrong.

—Plutarch

20

Back and Neck Pain— Why?

We sit at breakfast, we sit on the train on the way to work, we sit at lunch, we sit all afternoon . . . a hodge-podge of sagging livers, sinking gallbladders, drooping stomachs, compressed intestines, and squashed pelvic organs.

—John Button, Jr.

Sitting is also very tough on your back and neck. Back and neck pain are common, and can be very painful. Although often mistaken for a mysterious, permanent, unavoidable condition, back and neck pain are almost always easily treated, and more easily prevented.

Why read this if your back or neck don't hurt? Odds are they will one day. Statistically 8 out of 10 backs and necks over the age of 18 will hurt a little, a lot, or an awful lot sometime in their lives. Only the common cold beats back pain as the top cause of work absenteeism in the United States. Americans lose an estimated 90 million production days annually. Back injuries are the work industry's single greatest medical expense, estimated at $100 billion in the United States alone in medical costs, compensation, and lost productivity and wages— every year.

An Injury, Not a Condition

The real cause of most back and neck pain may surprise you. Just like heart disease and lung cancer, back and neck pain usually develop slowly over time without your knowing it. Back and neck pain are almost always a repetitive strain-type injury, not an unavoidable, sudden "condition," or evolutionary punishment for walking on two legs. This is an important distinction. Your chronic backache, your killer back-of-the-neck pain, or the back that just "goes out" once in a while are injuries that usually develop slowly from harmful patterns—things that you do every day.

Someone who breaks his leg would not go around year after year saying he has "leg condition." Back pain is an injury that can be treated, not a "condition" that cannot be changed.

Just as after a sprained ankle or broken arm, you can heal from back pain and resume your normal life. The key is to identify and modify abusive patterns, detailed in the next chapter on treating and preventing back and neck pain. First, a quick look at your interesting anatomy, so you can see why the things you do can hurt so much.

Just like heart disease and lung cancer, back and neck pain are usually developed slowly over time, from small, repetitive bad habits that cause injury. That means you can do something about it before it happens.

Your Interesting Parts

Your Spine Bones

The bones of your spine are called vertebrae. The top 7 vertebrae are your neck bones, called cervical vertebrae. Their names are C1 (from the top) down to C7. If you tip your head forward and feel the back of your neck, the bump at the bottom of your neck is usually C7. Your next 12 vertebrae are thoracic vertebrae (T1–T12). Your rib bones attach to these vertebrae, 12 on each side. (Both men and women have 12 paired ribs, 24 total. Men do not have one fewer rib, contrary to biblical speculation.) The next 5 vertebrae do not have ribs attached. These are your lower back bones, the lumbar vertebrae

(L1–L5). This is where a lot of back pain occurs. More on why in a bit. Below them are your 5 sacral vertebrae (S1–S5), fused into a single bone, the sacrum. The sacrum forms the bony back wall of your hips. Attached to the bottom of your sacrum is the coccyx, your tailbone.

C1-C7
Cervical
Vertebrae

T1-T12
Thoracic
Vertebrae

L1-L5
Lumbar
Vertebrae

Sacral
Vertebrae

Figure 20.1. You normally have 7 neck vertebrae (cervical); 12 upper back vertebrae (thoracic); 5 low back vertebrae (lumbar); 5 sacral vertebrae, fused into the bony back wall of your pelvis; and your small tailbone or coccyx, made of several fused rudimentary vertebrae.

Your Discs

Discs are flat, fibrocartilage cushions that sit like washers between bones in several areas of your body. The discs you hear about most often sit between each of your vertebrae. These intervertebral discs cushion shocks transmitted through your spine with your every step, and prevent your vertebrae from rubbing directly against each other.

There are also discs in other areas of your body. Tiny little discs cushion the joint between your head bone, called the temporal bone, and your lower jawbone, called the mandible. Sometimes these little discs wear out, causing pain at the joint between them, the temporo-mandibular joint (TMJ). You have two larger discs, called menisci (singular is meniscus), in each knee. Injuring a meniscus is one cause of knee pain.

The discs most often involved in low back pain are your vertebral discs between L4 and L5 and, particularly, between L5 and S1. That is where most people give the most punishment to their backs. Here's why.

The Quick Way and the Slow Way to Get Back and Neck Pain

There are two main ways to hurt your back and neck: the quick way and the slow way.

The Quick Way

The most classic onset of back pain is after you lean over, twist to the side, and lift something. Why is this?

If you do nothing more than stand still and bend over with straight legs, you put hundreds of pounds of force on each vertebral disc, the most on L5–S1. Twisting when you lean is worse. Yanking a weight is often the death blow. There are many opportunities to do exactly those three things: picking up packages and children, lifting things out of cars and trunks, making beds, taking out the trash, doing laundry, and grabbing your bags at the airport baggage area.

It's not that lifting by itself is bad for you. Lifting properly is no problem and can be good for you. Lots of people lift weights as a hobby or to make a living. Many people even lift dangerously for years without outward sign of injury—until one day . . .

The Slow Way

Years of wear and tear add up. Chronic slouching can injure your back and neck over several years as badly as you could in a single accident. Your body weight alone is enough to injure your muscle and discs through poor sitting, standing, and bending habits.

The small of your back is supposed to curve inward to a certain extent. One of several ways to slowly hurt your low back involves reversing your normal slight inward curve so that you curve forward

Figure 20.2. The quick way to ruin your back—lean over, twist, and lift.

instead, like the letter "C." This bad posture involves a motion called lumbar flexion.

The pressure of your own body weight on your muscles and discs over several years of poor posture is enough to injure your back as badly as a single accident.

Flexion is when you bend a joint to make it smaller. Bending your elbow is elbow flexion. Putting your chin on your chest is neck flexion. You do hip flexion when you bend forward at the hip or raise your leg. Genuflection (*genu* is the Latin word for "knee") is when you bend your knee in church, but it's just plain knee flexion any other time. Sitting, standing, and lifting with a round back instead of maintaining the normal inward curve of your lower back is lumbar flexion. Too much lumbar flexion squeezes and pushes your discs outward toward the back. The disc may eventually fray and give out like a worn tire. Continuous back flexion also overstretches the long ligament down the back of your spine, weakening the back and allowing discs more room to protrude. On top of that, chronically holding back muscles, or any muscles for that matter, in a stretched position weakens them.

Habitually standing with your head forward overstretches and "uncurves" the back of your neck with similar results. A forward head contributes to upper back pain, usually between the shoulders, just under the lower point of the shoulder blade, and may also radiate to other areas.

Figure 20.3. Normal good posture has a small inward curve in your low back. Chronically reversing your normal curve with poor posture can lead to back problems.

One of several ways to slowly hurt your back is sitting and bending so that the normal inward curve of your lower back curves outward. This eventually pushes discs outward and overstretches the long ligament down the back of the spine, weakening your back and allowing discs more room to protrude.

The second main bad posture is caused by weak abdominal muscles that allow your low back to sway backwards, exaggerating the normal inward curve. This does not cancel out problems from excess flexion, but creates back pain of its own. Often people who sit and bend with too much back flexion also stand excessively arched. Too much arching can cause the same wear-and-tear problems as too much flexion. Occasionally, too much arching irritates the joints, called vertebral facets, where each vertebra attaches to the one above and below it.

According to some estimates, men suffer back pain two to three times more often than women. One reason is the load of carrying around their larger shoulders, bigger backs, and longer, larger torsos relative to their bodies, than women. Women usually keep more of their weight lower and biomechanically safer.

Figure 20.4. Chronically exaggerating and forcing the normal inward curve of your low back is a poor posture that can lead to back pain.

Most people unknowingly abuse their backs all the time in their daily activities. Just as smoking one cigarette at a time eventually can cause much trouble, you can gradually accumulate a back injury that may not become apparent for years.

In an average day, most people repeatedly abuse their backs unknowingly. In this way they are brewing a back injury that may not become apparent for years. Ironically, once their backs finally begin to hurt, they give up active exercise that helps backs, and they continue sitting and lifting with a rounded back, and standing with too much arch—both major back injury–producing actions. A particularly ironic sight is back pain patients in physicians' and physical therapy waiting rooms, sitting in lumbar flexion and worsening their condition while they sit. What follows is a series of seemingly harmless daily habits that are continuous, major back and neck pain producers.

An Average Day of Ruining Your Back and Neck

You wake up and sit at the edge of the bed, curled in back and neck flexion. Then you slouch over to the sink and bend over the sink to splash your face awake. Bend over, twist, and lift to make the bed. Get dressed, bending wrong to pull on shoes and socks. Put a wallet in your back pocket that makes you sit crooked. Sit curled forward in lumbar and neck flexion in a kitchen chair, then again in the car or public transit to work. Commuting healthy by bicycle? Back flexion there too, worse with racing handlebars, if you curl over them in poor form. You add to your neck troubles when you crane your neck forward for the ride. Sit in flexion at work including lunch. From your chair, lean over, twist, and yank open file cabinets. Crane your neck forward at your desk to view the computer monitor. If your computer monitor is in the usual low position on your desk, you hold your head both forward and down to get your work done. Stand and walk with excess back arching (and also a forward head, often carrying packages which compounds the strain). Commute home sitting in flexion.

Maybe to the gym? Several popular exercises do more to weaken your back than strengthen it: weight lifting while leaning over unsupported, straight-leg dead lifting, forced repetitive back bending like toe touches from a stand, or swinging elbows down to opposite knees, and forced repetitive back arching like "donkey kicks" that swing the leg overhead from a hands-and-knees position.

Well-meaning exercisers often start their routine with a back abuse doozie—they bend over straight legged to touch toes, worse with bouncing and without warm-up. Although it often feels good on tight muscles, it's tough on your back in the long run. Moreover, stretching is not a warm-up, and should not be done until you warm yourself by muscular activity like jogging or bicycling. Necks get yanked forward during sit-ups, crunches, and several other exercises involving the hands behind the head and pulling the upper body forward. Chest exercises shorten and strengthen the upper chest muscles, while upper back muscles are ignored, furthering the rounded shoulder-forward head posture problem. Properly trained exercise instructors know not to do these exercises, but exercises that produce back and neck pain are still remarkably widespread in gyms and schools across the country. Healthy alternatives are in Chapter 8, "What Exercises Do You Need to Be Fit?" and Chapter 9, "Good and Bad Exercises."

Do you use rowing machines? Rowing machines can be terrific exercise when done correctly, but problematic when done incorrectly with a rounded back. Sit upright, keeping the lower natural inward curve of your low back. Push off your heels, rather than your toes to get better exercise for your legs.

Still doing sit-ups not crunches? Still doing leg raises? Those two do little for your abdominal muscles and are tough on your lower back, specifically where the muscles you use for sit-ups and leg lifts connect. *See* Chapter 7 on abdominal muscles for a detailed explanation of why sit-ups and leg lifts benefit other muscles more than your abs, and what to do instead.

Finished your workout? Bend over and twist to pick up your gym bag and sling it over one shoulder. A paper on "Asymmetrical Loads and Lateral Bending of the Human Spine" in the July 1993 *Medical & Biological Engineering and Computing* reported that loads like bags worn over one shoulder curl your spine slightly. The researchers concluded that such unequal forces might contribute to the high percentage of school children turning up with scoliosis. They suggested switching to knapsacks to distribute the load. In adults, shoulder bags seem to contribute to muscular pain.

Flexion for your commute home, at dinner, in front of the sink, and in a rounded chair or couch in front of the TV with your head craned forward. Have young kids? Bend over wrong to pick them up. Hold them while standing arched. Flexion to tuck them in. Add chronic incorrect lifting during house and yard work.

This overview just scratches the surface of what's behind back pain but you get the idea. Just like braces on your teeth, the continuous push of bad posture habits on your back and neck will eventually reshape your body in unhealthy ways. Major factors in this process are weak muscles, lack of flexibility, poor sitting, standing, and bending habits. It's not just lifting wrong one day. The effects are cumulative, like smoking. Then, one day you bend over to pick up a sock and your back bids you *"hastalumbago."*

The relentless pull of bad posture habits all day, every day, on your back and neck, will eventually reshape them, just like braces on your teeth, Only the result is not pretty or healthy.

The Details on How You Usually Get Back and Neck Pain

This section does not deal with special cases of pain from arthritis, osteoporosis, or scoliosis. However, the bad habits described here

Figure 20.5. An average day of slowly ruining your back with poor posture starts in the morning and goes on all day, every day, for many people. You don't hurt your back from lifting wrong once. It is from things you do all the time without realizing it. Like smoking, the ill effects take years to accumulate.

increase anyone's risk of pain and injury. For more on osteoporosis origins and prevention *see* Chapter 22, "Calcium, Protein, Space Flight, Exercise, and Your Bones—A Detective Story."

Muscles

Most back and neck pain is muscle-related. There are several ways you contribute to this happening:

- Ordinary daily bad habits, like chronic poor sitting, standing, and bending habits, eventually overstretch, strain, and contract your muscles into painful knots.
- Bad posture puts your head and torso into positions that put relentless pressure on discs, nerves, and muscles. Micro tears, spasm, and inflammation result, creating more pain.
- Sometimes muscles on one side of your spine or hip are stronger than the muscles on the other side. The weaker side can't counter the pull of stronger opposing muscles, furthering bad posture stress.
- Sometimes muscles on one side of your spine or hip are too tight compared to the balancing muscles on the other side, pulling your body into a continuing cycle of poor posture and joint stress.
- Tight muscles can strain instead of stretch during activity. Even a small range of motion can strain tight low back muscles, accounting for many painful backs at the end of a day.
- Muscle strength and flexibility inequalities can occur even in people who work out regularly, if they don't work muscle groups evenly, a common practice.
- Muscles called hip flexors bend your leg forward at the hip. One set of hip flexor muscles begins on your lumbar vertebrae (lower back bones) and extends forward and down to a knob on your upper leg bone (the greater trochanter of your femur). When these muscles are tight, common in people who sit a lot, it sometimes pulls enough on your lower back to increase its normal arch. This extra pulling and tilting can contribute to low back pain.
- Other sets of muscles pull on your hipbones from the back. Hamstrings are the triple set of muscles in the back of your thigh. They work to both bend your knee and swing your leg behind you. The three hamstrings of each leg start at the bottom of your hipbones, on the bony "bumps" you sit on, called ischial tuberosities. The hamstrings run down the back of each leg, and cross the back of your knee where you can feel their stringy tendons on both sides. Tight hamstrings are thought to pull enough on the hipbones to tip the pelvis rearward, reversing your normal arch and contributing to back pain.
- Muscles that are tight from inflexibility, and muscles that are tightly in spasm from bad posture habits, can compress nerves, mimicking the kind of pain produced by herniated discs press-

Figure 20.6. Your hip flexor muscles cross your hip in the front and attach to the top of your leg. They work to bend (flex) your hip joint. One set of your hip flexors starts on your spine, the others on the top of your hip. Tight hip flexors can change the way you stand and walk, and contribute to back pain.

ing on nerves. One of several muscles that seems to like to do this is the piraformis muscle. The piraformis lies deep in your pelvis under your buttock muscles. In a small percentage of the population, the sciatic nerve goes through the piraformis. In most others, the sciatic nerve is not in the piraformis, but close by. In either case, if the piraformis is tight, it can compress your sciatic nerve, causing pain and sometimes weakness in the buttock and down your leg.

Tight hip, back, and leg muscles can cause the poor
postures that lead to back and neck pain.

Any of these various muscle problems are often enough to cause back pain by themselves. Worse, several of them frequently occur together. Add slinging weights and packages (or yourself) around in ways your back isn't designed to withstand, and back pain eventually afflicts the majority of people.

Most back and neck pain comes from daily bad sitting, standing, and bending postures.

What About Your Neck? Poor neck posture often brings on pain, and sometimes even numbness in the back of your head, down the side of your neck, across the top of your shoulders, between the shoulders, under the shoulder blades, and sometimes down your arm. Poor neck posture is a common cause of headache.

The most common poor neck posture is standing and sitting with your neck sloped forward, which juts your head forward of the center line of your body. This bad posture is called a forward head. Many people have a forward head without knowing it. Think of a bowling ball. Now imagine continuously holding that heavy bowling ball out in front of your body. Soon, your back and neck muscles that hold it will fatigue, then hurt. That bowling ball is your head.

A forward head looks like E.T. sniffing a flower. Less comical is its effect to overstretch the ligament down the back of your neck, putting pressure on your discs. A forward head can eventually damage neck and upper back structures, when they begin to bend and rub at angles they were not built for. Your discs can degenerate or begin to protrude. Protruding (herniated) discs can press on nerves that go down your arms. Chronically holding your neck muscles, or any muscles, in an overstretched position weakens them. You wind up with shortened contracted muscles down the front of your neck, and a stretched weakened upper back. You may have seen this forward head posture on older people and wondered how they got that way. The answer is—practice.

The forward head can also contribute to shoulder trouble. The forward head posture brings the top of the shoulder bone over the top of the arm bone, limiting overhead reaching, and over time, contributing to shoulder impingement problems.

An average day is filled with opportunities for the bad habit of the forward head:

- Sitting with your head craning forward in front of the computer screen.
- Hunching over your desk.
- Using your shoulder to cradle a phone receiver against your ear.

Figure 20.7. A forward head can cause a lot of neck, shoulder, and upper back pain. A forward head can make you look older. A forward head is so common that it looks normal, and is just about taken for granted in older people. But it is a posture that can be avoided.

- Commuting in car, bus, or train seats.
- Bending over the kids.
- While walking.
- While doing household chores.
- Watching TV.
- Craning your head forward while exercising.

In short: All day, every day, at work and play, even at rest in a chair, and then all night if you sleep on your back with your head pushed forward with pillows. No wonder your neck and back are killing you.

The average person does so many things every day to
damage their back and neck, that it is amazing that
their back and neck doesn't hurt more often.

Discs

Disc protrusions, called herniations, can result from chronic outward pressure on discs. In your neck and lower back, this pressure occurs from the bad posture of slouching your torso forward into the shape of the letter "C" when sitting, bending, and lifting, rather than keeping the normal inward curves of the neck and lower back. Continually putting grinding, unequal pressures on your discs can cause them to break down (degenerate) over time. The curled posture also pushes discs out, out, out, over time. The edges begin to fray like a wearing tire. Eventually, one day, after even a small provocation, the disc finally protrudes far enough for a sudden onset of disc pain. Then you attribute the injury of the "slipped disc" to the one event that brought on the pain, never realizing it was brewing all along from the way you sat, stood, and lifted, day after day, year after year.

Year after year of poor sitting and standing posture can wear out your discs. One day, a disc finally "goes," even doing nothing more than sneezing or reaching for something. The "slipped disc" wasn't from the one event; it was brewing all along.

Discs don't usually protrude straight back. Their path is blocked by a long, tough, vertically running ligament, called the posterior longitudinal ligament. That is good because your spinal cord lies behind the discs. But that also means that a disc herniation will usually push out sideways. The long nerves serving your legs also exit your lumbar vertebrae to the side. When a disc bulges against these nerves, pain extends down your leg. The most common nerve to be pushed on by "slipping" discs is the sciatic nerve. The sciatic nerve has both sensory and motor functions, meaning that if compressed, it will hurt and can reduce the function of your leg. In the most serious cases, discs can protrude directly backwards against your spine, disrupting your ability to move from that level down, and control your bowel and bladder.

Although "slipped" or herniated discs used to be thought of as a life sentence, we now know that is rarely so. Many disc protrusions heal if you let them, and you can go back to your life, as after any other injury. Chapter 21, next, covers treating and preventing muscle- and disc-related back and neck pain. It's not hard, and rarely requires surgery. Best of all, back and neck pain, whether from muscle or disc, is almost always avoidable.

Most disc herniations will heal with proper exercises and stopping the bad habits that made them herniate in the first place.

Neck and Back Pain from Other Parts of Your Body

Your Legs

A knee or ankle injury may throw off how you walk and stand. Poor posture of your legs, which causes you to distribute your weight unevenly across your legs and feet, can affect how you walk, and adds to chronic wear and tear on your muscles and joints.

Unequal leg length can add to back pain. (It is a myth that everyone has unequal leg length.) For those who do have unequal leg lengths, the difference is not always truly in bone length. Sometimes muscle spasm can pull your hip and lower body out of normal alignment, making a "functional" leg length difference, rather than a true structural one. These spasms can be easily dealt with by a good physical therapist, orthopedist, physical medicine physician, osteopath, or massage therapist with appropriate training. If your doctor finds you have a true leg length difference, wear a properly measured, padded shoe lift that fits well.

Your Feet

An often overlooked source of back pain is the foot. You may walk with your feet too flat (pronated) or too arched. Or turned in or turned out. Bad foot posture throws off how your legs distribute your weight. Another foot problem may involve your big toe. When your big toe joint works as it should, it bends pliably, and your foot and leg pivot around it to walk normally. Sometimes, although it may not hurt or be obvious, it does not bend enough during the push-off phase of walking, throwing off foot position, gait, and pushing the posture of your head and trunk forward. Your lower back muscles and discs bear the brunt. For more on how important your feet can be in pain and injury prevention, and exercises to prevent problems, *see* Chapter 9.

Your Middle

The extra load and altered posture of beer guts and pregnancies is tough on your back.

Your Walk

Walking "hard" shocks your spine and adds to early wear and tear. Some people come down so heavily on each step that the skin on their face jiggles. Think of your car. Without good shock absorption, your car will wear out early. You have several ways to add to your necessary, natural shock absorption:

- Your major bodily shock absorbers are your thigh and backside muscles, the quadriceps and gluteal muscles. Exercise them for better back health.
- Strong back muscles are shock absorbers, much more so than weak back muscles, another good reason to do your back exercises.
- Wear a good, padded insole in your shoes every day. Two good brands of padded insoles are Spenco® and SecondWind®. When you buy new shoes, take your padded insoles with you and try them on in the shoe. If you have to buy a half size higher to fit the pad, it's worth it.
- Maintain good posture by keeping the normal inward curve of your lower back. Your spine is like a spring and absorbs shock through its normal curves. Straightening out the curve by slouching removes the normal spring action. Accentuating the normal curve through too much arching also reduces shock absorption.
- And of course, walk softly.

Your legs and feet have posture, too. How you stand and walk makes a big difference between getting healthy exercise, and putting extra pressures, shocks, and wear and tear on your joints.

Neck and Back Pain from Outside Your Body

Your Shoes

Shoes are often made with little or no shock absorption, particularly fashionable dress shoes. They are also frequently too tight for good walking dynamics, even if they do not feel too tight.

- If you have marks, bruises, roughness, or calluses on your foot or toes, chances are that your shoes are too tight.

- If your toes fit like puzzle pieces, tight shoes probably molded them that way.
- Tight shoes aggravate and accelerate bunion formation in people predisposed to them. Bunions alter healthy walking mechanics.
- High heels are well known as major contributors to foot injury and disruption of normal walking mechanics of the entire leg, transmitting problems to your back, and even to your neck.
- Worn-out shoes can create a vicious cycle. If you walk unevenly, your shoes wear unevenly. Turn your shoes over and look at the heels. See if they are much more worn down on one side than the other. This uneven sole will tilt you further to that side, making you walk even more unevenly.
- Walk straight, and keep the heels of your shoes in good repair. Don't wear old, poorly worn shoes.

It's a myth that sneakers don't have "support" or are bad for your feet. Dress shoes are more often the culprit. With practically nothing between the soles of your feet and the hard pavement, and raised heels that alter normal walking dynamics of the foot, it's a marvel that your back and neck don't hurt more often.

Good shock absorption is important to healthy backs and necks. Wear shoes with low or no heels, padded insoles, and soft soles.

Your Clothes

Tight pants and belts can make your back hurt.

Your Mattress

Too-hard mattresses are a common cause of tight, stiff morning backs. It is an "old husband's tale" that back pain sufferers must sleep on a hard board. Try a foam "egg crate" on top of your hard mattress.

Your Chair

Check your car seat. Does it make you sit curled forward? Is it worn out on one side, making you sit with one hip hiked higher than the other? Check your chair at work. Do you sit crooked? Maybe your seat is not level. Put your computer monitor up on blocks so that you look at it straight on, not craning your neck down and forward to view it at desk level. Check your chair height at your desk.

Your Cigarettes

Smoking contributes to degeneration of your discs.

Hidden Causes of Back and Neck Pain

The major, usual causes of back and neck pain are tight, weak back and leg muscles, a forward head posture, and poor standing and sitting postures. There are also surprising and often overlooked contributors to pain:

- Funny leg posture. Keep your knees facing straight ahead rather than letting them turn in or out. Keep them in line with your ankle joint, rather than letting them bow out or sag inward.
- Funny foot posture. Stand with your weight distributed evenly so that you do not roll in or out on your arches. Check your shoes to see if they make you stand funny.
- "Stuck" big toe. Your big toe needs to bend with each step so that you can push off your toe, rather than lifting the entire foot stiffly. Keep your feet flexible, particularly your big toe joint.
- Beer guts.
- Walking "hard." It shocks your spine and adds to early wear and tear.
- Not wearing sneakers often enough. Just like a car, you need good shock absorbers or your frame will show early wear.
- High heels—they alter just about everything natural about your foot, leg, and back posture, all the way to your neck.
- Old shoes that are unevenly worn, or new shoes that do not fit right so that your foot is allowed to or made to tilt to either side.
- Tight pants and belts.

- Too-hard mattresses.
- Chairs that make you sit funny.
- Computer monitors at desk level, rather than head level.
- Smoking—directly adds to disc degeneration.

Next—What to do about back and neck pain.

21

Back and Neck Pain— Prevention and Treatment

We don't consider a patient cured when his sprain has healed or he's restored to a minimal level of functioning. The patient is cured when he can again do the things he loves to do.

—Stanley A. Herring

The previous chapter described some of the easy, common ways to get back and neck pain. To review, back and neck pain often result from things you do every day without knowing it. Although back pain often comes on suddenly, the injury that causes pain is rarely a sudden event. It brews with years of abuse. Wear and tear from your body weight alone from poor sitting, standing, and bending habits can injure your back over time as badly as might happen in a single accident. The main factors in back and neck pain are poor sitting, standing, and lifting postures that often result from inflexibility and weakness of muscles supporting your torso and back. This can happen even if you work out regularly.

Most Back and Neck Pain Is Preventable

The Red Cross estimates that 90% of all back pain is preventable. You can easily reduce your chance of back or neck pain and reduce pain you already have. You first need to identify and avoid things you do that chronically abuse your back and neck. Then do several easy exercises to help you recover and make your back more injury resistant.

Even with things you can't prevent, such as certain inherited back disorders, or serious accidents, you can usually reduce or eliminate pain with good habits. A tendency toward arthritis, for example, increases with habits that contribute to wear and tear. Scoliosis may be aggravated by carrying shoulder bags, or skipping exercises to strengthen muscles that support the spine. There is much that you can control.

Almost all back pain is preventable.

Avoid Bad Standing, Sitting and Lifting Habits

Your Back

Do you sit, stand, and bend with your lower back rounded outward rather than inward? That is the most common way to slowly ruin your back. The concave back of most chairs makes you sit with a rounded back and a forward head. Watch for bad chair engineering in office, bus, train, and plane seats. Other problem chairs are bench seats in restaurants and church pews. Plane and bus seats seem to be exceptionally bad. Boat benches are often hard with no back at all. The stress to your back may be made worse when pounding over waves. When riding in trains, planes, and automobiles, bring a small cushion to place in the small of your back, to sit keeping the normal inward curve of your lower back.

Sitting stresses your discs more than standing. Poor sitting posture makes the strain far worse.

Do you stand with too much arch in your back? You might need abdominal exercises to increase the forward "guy wires" that can prevent too much backward sway.

Do you pick things up by bending at the waist with your legs straight or nearly so? Don't do that. Keep your torso upright, not bent over, and bend your knees. A common complaint is that using the legs is difficult. Exercise your leg muscles, discussed below, to make it easier. When you have one hand or elbow free, support your upper body weight with that hand or elbow on your knee or other support. Don't twist to one side during a lift or bend.

Your Neck

Do you stand and sit with your head forward? That's a common source of upper back, neck, and head pain, and particularly, pain between and across the shoulders. A forward head is so common that it looks normal, but is serious. Keep your ears over your shoulders, not in front of them. A common mistake is just lifting the chin up, which just compounds the pinching, rather than pulling it back and in. Put your computer monitor up on blocks, rather than sitting it on the desk, so that you can look at it straight on without looking down. Place your TV screen at head level. Reading and writing at a desk is no excuse to hunch over. Keep your body upright, and head pulled back while you look down, rather than tipping your head down and forward.

Figure 21.1. Correct a forward head by lifting up and in, so that your ears line up over the center of your shoulders. Look forward, not up or down. This is also a good exercise to relieve pain and tension in your neck and shoulders.

Relieving back and neck pain does not mean giving up activities you love, or sitting and standing stiffly like a soldier. You need physical activity and flexible posture.

Your "Guy Wires"

Your back needs support from all sides. In brief, muscles running along your back keep a certain amount of pull on the back of your spine all the time to keep you from slouching over forward. Abdominal muscles, which run down your front from your ribs to your pelvic bones, pull similarly to keep you from arching too far backward during normal standing and sitting. Weakness in your guy wire muscles allow you to sit and stand in positions that slowly injure you without being aware of it. The degree of strength and muscular endurance of your back muscles can make the difference between an uneventful day, and a tired, achy back that night. That's why back exercises are so important.

Figure 21.2. Your abdominal muscles are your 'guy wires' that support your spine from the front, and your back muscles are your 'guy wires' in the back. Weak guy wire muscles allow you to sit and stand in poor postures that can slowly cause back and neck pain.

Avoid Too Little Exercise

Without enough exercise, your back muscles easily become weak. Weak muscles can't hold the good posture necessary for anatomic structures to fit together without strain and rubbing. This can happen even if you are in "good shape" or go to the gym. It is easy to underwork some muscles, and overwork others so that they overpower the back and neck muscles.

Avoid Too Much Exercise of the Wrong Kind

Several exercises common at gyms and exercise studios can do your back more harm than good. A few bad exercises now and then usually does little damage, but give it a chance. Like smoking, the repeated damage of the exposure can harm at a rate faster than your body can repair.

Tough-on-the-Back Exercises

- Straight-legged dead lifting. You hear all the time never to lean over and lift packages with straight legs, so why does it magically become all right to do that in a gym? Many lifters believe it strengthens the back, but straight-legged dead lifting can injure you.
- Repeated bouncing on toe touches. It is just more leaning over with straight legs with the added stress of the quick, repeated strain on the back.

It's well known that you should never lean over and lift packages with straight legs, so why does it magically become all right to do that in a gym? Straight-legged dead lifting can seriously injure your back.

- Sit-ups and leg lifts (unless you need them for activities requiring high hip flexor strength, like ballet, place kicking, and martial arts). Sit-ups and leg lifts use the hip flexor muscles that attach to your lower spine, far more than they use your abdominal muscles. They are tough on the back with little reward for the abs. Substitute crunches, described in Chapter 7 on abdominal muscles.

- Forced, repetitive back arching that, over the years, can irritate your facet joints, where each vertebrae joins the next. Examples are continuously swinging your leg backwards in the air in an exercise called "donkey kicks," and by standing with too much arch, particularly when lifting weights overhead. With better fitness education, these problematic exercises are slowly being replaced with safer techniques, but they are still common.

Abs Are Not Enough

Many people mistakenly concentrate on abdominal exercises like crunches, thinking that these alone will keep their backs injury free. It is all too common for exercise classes to spend much time on abdominal exercises, and never turn over to do back exercises. Without also working the back muscles, you can strengthen your "abs" until your relatively weaker back muscles can't counter the pull from the front. The resulting forward slouch slowly injures. Abs create an important support structure for your torso, but they are not the entire support. Back exercises are detailed, in a bit.

To Avoid Back and Neck Pain, Avoid These:

- Continuous incorrect lifting, sitting and standing.
- Sitting with your lower back rounded.
- Continually holding your head forward.
- Chronic bending at the waist.
- Twisting during a lift or bend.
- Damaging exercises.
- Beer guts.
- High heels.
- Smoking.
- Lack of exercise.
- Poor flexibility of back, hip, and hamstrings.
- Doing ab exercises without turning over to counter them with back exercises.

Posture Matters More Than You Think

Posture can make a difference between a pain-free back and neck, and chronic misery. Keep your ears over the center line of your shoulders. Keep your shoulders centered over your hips, hips over knee joints, and knee joints over ankle joints. Not stiffly, but naturally. The fitness of your supporting musculature will determine whether you can maintain good posture, or slouch and crane into postures that eventually will be a pain in the neck or behind. How can you tell?

Posture Test

To identify how your body segments line up:

- Stand very near a wall, facing away from the wall, but not touching it.
- Assume a posture that you feel is normal.
- Carefully, slowly, back up and contact the wall.
- Did your head, shoulders, back, behind, calves, and heels all touch at once? Good posture. Did your behind touch first? You probably slouch forward. You need to concentrate on the back muscles that support your posture upright by pulling toward the back. Did your shoulders touch first? You might be arching backwards and need extra abdominal muscle strengthening to keep your "guy wires" supporting you from the front. Did the back of your head never touch? You probably have a forward head.

If you habitually keep your head forward of your shoulders, then learn to correct that by pulling your chin in. Don't just tip your chin up. Slide the head back until it can touch the wall with the rest of your body when you do your posture checks (a good habit to get in to). Try it for ten counts, then hold all day.

Watch other people from the side as they stand, walk, and sit, so that you can identify a forward head. At home, spend time to learn about your own posture. Stand sideways in front of a mirror. Use a second, hand-held mirror to look at your profile, or use a three-way mirror. See where your ears are relative to the middle of your shoulder. See where your shoulder is relative to your back and hips, and so on.

Figure 21.3. Try a posture test by slowly backing up against a wall. Did your behind touch first? Or your shoulders? Did the back of your head never touch? Line up all your segments comfortably. Then keep that good posture all day. Posture can make a difference between a pain-free back and neck, and chronic misery.

Many people feel "unnatural" standing with good posture.
Others say they need to "relax" by slouching.
When the postural muscles of your back and abdomen
get so weak and tight that they cannot comfortably
support you, that means you need to work them to be
comfortable, not slouch to be comfortable.

Posture Exercise

Many people have such tight muscles in front, and such stretch-weakened muscles in back, that standing up straight feels uncomfortable, tiring, and unnatural. Being unable to maintain upright posture comfortably is a signal of the simple but important exercises that need to be done. The "wall stand" posture exercise helps you identify and relearn good posture:

- Stand against a wall with your heels, behind, shoulders, and the back of your head all touching the wall at once.
- Look straight forward and hold. Don't force back or stand rigidly like a soldier. Just hold your body upright.

- Pull your shoulders back—not until they hurt, but until the midline of your shoulder matches the midline of your body, not in front of it. Your back may be touching the wall, but your shoulders may still be rounded forward.
- You may need to stretch your chest a bit to allow your shoulders to line up with the midline of your body, rather than rounding forward.
- Get the feel of this correct posture, then try to do it as a habit.
- Do this every 15 minutes or so when you are spending time sitting in a chair or leaning over work on a table.

Healthy Sitting Posture

When you sit in a chair or in the car, use a lumbar roll:

- Keep a small rolled towel or commercially available lumbar roll between your lower back and the chair. The roll will support you in a healthy, inward-curved lumbar posture.
- You don't need to force your body into an unnaturally straight or arched posture. Just relax against the roll.
- Keep one lumbar roll in the car and one at your desk. Carry a roll in your bag or briefcase for unexpected meetings or movies. If you find yourself without your lumbar roll, press a rolled towel, article of clothing, or even your arm into service.
- Commercially available rolls are sometimes too fat. An easy solution for those made of foam is to cut them in half lengthwise, making two long rolls, each round on one surface and flat on the opposite. Put the flat part against the chair and the rounded side to the small of your back.

Healthy Work Habits

You can do many healthy things for your back during the day:

- When working at your desk, remember to stand up every half hour or so and arch your back in the other direction.
- Chores are no excuse to slouch and reverse your lumbar curve. When cleaning, painting, or fixing, bend your knees rather than curl over the task. Keep your torso upright, and preserve the natural inward curve of your back.

Figure 21.4. Use a lumbar roll when you sit, to keep the normal inward curve of your low back. Make a lumbar roll from a small cushion, a rolled towel, or cut a cylindrical foam roll into two half-rolls for a custom fit.

- After bicycling, gardening, cleaning floors, or any other activity where you lean forward for prolonged periods (even with bent knees and good posture), lie facedown, propped up on your elbows so that your back curves backwards.
- When stuck sitting for long periods, during movies or traveling, do small range of motion stretches. Alternately tense and release your leg, back, and torso muscles. Press your palms firmly against your thighs. Press your palms firmly against the back of your head, and push back with your neck. Keep breathing during all exercises.
- Any time you find yourself bending forward for long periods, counter it with leaning backward.

Doing your back exercises a few times a week, but keeping
the old, bad postures and habits that hurt in your back
in the first place is like eating cake and ice cream morning,
noon, and night, and doing 5 minutes of aerobics a few times
a week. You are not balancing out the harm done.

Healthy Lifting Habits

Any time you bend over, whether for a drink of water, to wash your face in the sink, to tie your shoe, or to lift your packages, bend your knees. It's not wimpy. It will save your back from cumulative abuse that it was not built to withstand. When lifting anything heavy or light:

- Get close and face the weight.
- Keep your feet apart.
- Bend your knees.
- Keep your torso upright.
- Take a deep breath.
- Think "I don't want to hurt my back" *before* you just lean over and yank.
- Lift slowly.

Figure 21.5. Safe lifting technique. Keep your torso upright, get close and face the weight, bend your knees keeping your feet apart, and lift slowly. Do this any time you lift, whether for laundry, packages, or in the gym to get weights off the rack or floor.

If you lift dumbbells for back strength, don't bend over and lift. Lie on a flat or tilted bench, facedown. If you choose to stand, support your weight with one hand on a bench or your knee. You hear all the time not to bend over and lift anything because it's bad for your back, yet when people go to a gym, they magically forget this, and bend over and lift weights, thinking it will help their backs.

Safe Lifting with Bad Knees

Many people use the excuse of bad knees to lift things straight-legged. Bad knees are no excuse to make your back bad, too. If your knees hurt, go to a good orthopedist to find out why. Many knee complaints result over time just like back and neck pain—from poor walking and standing habits that wear, tear, and unevenly load the knee joint, and from uneven muscle strength and flexibility. Get your knees properly diagnosed, then do the knee exercises your doctor or physical therapist prescribes to make your knees better (knees are for another book).

Use the "golfer's pickup" to bend over:

- Put one foot in back of the other.
- Put your hand on your thigh.
- Lean your weight on your hand.
- Bend your knees as much as comfortable, keeping the weight of your upper body supported.

Try it now for practice.

Figure 21.6. Use the "golfer's pick-up" when picking up small things. You protect your back by supporting your upper body weight on your knee, and reduce stress on your knees by keeping a wide stance.

Healthy Standing Around

Whether standing in line, talking with people, or doing dishes, you can do several, easy, quick maneuvers to help your back:

- Check your back posture and correct it—are you arching too much or slouching so that you are removing the inward curve of your low back?
- Check your neck posture and correct it. Is your head forward? Pull it back in.
- Stand with one foot supported. That's why bars have that rail at shin level. At the kitchen sink, you can open the under-sink door and rest your foot on the shelf.
- Tuck your hips and pelvis in to stretch your back.
- Alternately tense and relax your ab, leg, and back muscles.
- Press your palms firmly against your thighs to work your torso muscles.

Healthy Exercises

Unfortunately, back pain is sometimes regarded the way a heart attack was years ago—as a condition, not an injury. Both were relegated to the "cardiac cripple" status of inactivity; never to exercise or lift weights, and even to restrict activities of daily living. In that way, a tragic cycle of disuse and declining ability perpetuates. Back muscles, like heart muscles, need exercise to develop in progressive sane ways until they meet your needs. Increased endurance of posture muscles of the back reduces back and knee pain over a long day. Increased strength reduces your chance of hurting your back, knees, and shoulders from lifting packages and weights. *See* Chapter 3, "Improving Your Fitness," for more on increasing muscle endurance and strength.

If you have back and/or neck pain, the exercises you need to do will be specific for the type of pain. There are many exercises that strengthen and stretch the hips, back, neck, abdominal muscles, and leg muscles, to reduce back and neck pain. See your physician or physical therapist before starting any exercise program, particularly if you have existing pain.

Neck Exercises

One exercise that corrects a forward head is called the "double-chin" exercise. Pull your head back into proper alignment in an exaggerated way, so that your chin becomes a "double chin." Hold for ten counts, release, and repeat.

Abdominal Exercises

Abdominal exercises are covered in Chapter 7. Strong abdominal muscles are important to support your torso from swaying backward. Exercises that contract your back muscles are crucial to complete the support your back needs to keep from slouching forward. These important back exercises are described next.

Upper Back Extension (also good for your neck)

1. Lie facedown, hands at your sides and off the floor. Slowly lift your upper body a few inches. This action is called back extension. Then lower back to the floor. Don't force. Start with one or two lifts. See how you feel the next day. If pain free, gradually increase to ten repetitions three times a week.
2. To progress, do more repetitions, and move your arms from your sides to overhead.
3. If you have a bench, lie on the bench facedown, and let your feet touch the floor. When you lift your torso, lift until your back is straight, rather than arched.

Figure 21.7. Upper back extension strengthens your upper back muscles, important for posture and back pain control. Don't yank or force upwards, but lift your arms and upper body with control.

Lower Back Extension

There are several ways to contract the muscles of your low back to exercise them:

1. Lie facedown, chin on hands. Lift one leg off the floor. Hold and lower. Easy does it. Then switch legs.
2. To progress, lift both legs together. This exercise is great for your behind as well.

3. If you have a low bench, lie on the bench facedown, and let your feet touch the floor. Lift your legs until your back is straight, rather than arched.

Figure 21.8. Lower back extension strengthens your lower back muscles, important for posture and back pain control. One way to do lower back extension is to lie facedown on the floor or over a bench, and gently lift one or both legs.

4. Lie on your back, both knees bent. Lift your behind off the floor and hold for ten seconds, then lower. Work up to ten repetitions. To progress to a harder variation, do this with only one leg. Cross one ankle over the opposite knee, or just hold one foot off the floor, and lift your hips.

Figure 21.9. Here is another way to strengthen your low back and gluteal muscles.

5. If you go to a gym that has weight machines, look for the back machine. You sit with a pad against your back and curl it backward. It should be next to the abdominal machine (where you sit with a pad against your abdomen and curl it forward). In a physical therapy setting, these machines will have special locks that limit how far you can push backwards. As your back gets better, the lock is moved to allow more range of motion.

This limit to motion is important during physical therapy of injured backs. Check with your doctor before using machines if you have a back injury.

Figure 21.10. Exercise to contract your back muscles is crucial for back health, good posture, and pain control. Remember the back machine when you use the ab machine.

Modifications for Special Populations

Some people with specific back disorders like facet pain and a slippage of vertebrae called spondylolisthesis (spon-di-lo-lis-THEE-sis) should not actively arch their back. However, contracting the back muscles is crucial to strengthening. For these conditions, exercises that contract the back muscles without arching past the neutral-straight position have been found to be useful and important for rehabilitation and pain control. Physical therapy centers and many gyms have back machines that allow active back extension while limiting the range to not exceed the straight position.

If you have been told that you shouldn't extend your back past the straight position, you can still exercise your back muscles in several ways.

- For your upper back, one easy exercise without arching your back is to lie facedown on the floor or over a bench, and lift only your arms, not your upper body.
- For your lower back, lean over a chair and lift one leg in back. If you have a bench, you can lie on the bench, so that the bench extends from your chin to your hips, with your legs

hanging freely to the floor. Then lift one or both legs up from the floor until your body is straight.

- Kneel on all fours on a soft mat. Raise one leg until it is straight behind you. At the same time, lift your opposite arm in front of you. Hold.

Figure 21.11. Some people with specific back disorders do better with modified back exercises.

Surprising Back Exercises

Push-ups are surprisingly good for your back. They use a lot of back and abdominal stabilization just holding the "ready" position. Even if you are not able to do push-ups, hold the ready position.

Therapeutic rubber tubes can be used for great back exercises. Secure the middle of a long rubber tube around a doorknob or other device at waist height. Hold both ends in front of you and stand far enough back that you create the desired tension on the band. Pull both arms straight down to your sides and hold. Repeat. You contract all your torso-stabilizing muscles for this one. Now with both arms still straight, lift both arms up overhead and hold. Repeat. Keep breathing.

Healthy Stretches

Good range of motion in all directions helps prevent back pain. Warm up before you stretch. Warm up means just as it sounds. Raise your body temperature. Slow jogging, bicycling, or anything that gets you to break a light sweat will make stretching safer. *See* Chapter 5 on warm-ups. See your physician before attempting any back exercises and for a back exercise program that suits your own back health.

Hamstring and Lower Back Stretches

Leaning over at the waist for toe touches does stretch your back and hamstrings, but it is not the best stretch for regular use. Although it often feels good on tight muscles, it's tough on your back in the long run. A safer back stretch is to lie on your back and stretch one leg at a time by holding it straight in the air and pulling it gently toward you.

A variation of this stretch, where the bent knee is pressed to the chest, produced an injury reported in the March 1993 *New England Journal of Medicine*. A compression injury named "stretcher's scrotum" occurred when a man performing the stretch wore restrictive gym shorts, squeezing the testes between the bent leg and the body. The *Journal* cautioned that practitioners prescribing such stretches for back pain should recommend that males wear loose, stretchable pants. Another good hamstring stretch is to stand with one heel propped up on a chair keeping the inward curve of your lower back, and sticking your behind out a little.

Figure 21.12. Here are two good stretches for your hamstrings without bending over from a stand, which is tough on your back. When doing this stretch standing, keep your back upright in normal alignment, rather than bent over forward.

Hip Flexor Stretches

Hip flexors, the muscles that bend your hip and raise your leg, as in walking, were covered in detail in Chapter 6 on stretching, and

Chapter 7 on abdominal muscles. Tight, short hip flexors are common. Hip flexor stretches are important to back health, but unfortunately neglected.

An easy way to stretch your hip flexors is the lunge. The lunge is often done improperly so that there is little or no stretch on the hip flexors. To do it properly, stand with your feet comfortably apart, then slide one foot in back of you as far as you can do comfortably. The trick is to not lean forward, and not arch backward, but tuck your behind under you. You will feel the stretch in your forward leg where it normally creases in front, in an area about the size of a small pancake.

Figure 21.13. The lunge is a good hip flexor stretch for the back leg. Avoid leaning forward or you won't stretch your back leg, but can stress your forward knee. Stand upright and tuck your behind inward.

Back Stretches

Many exercise programs concentrate on bending forward, forward, and more forward. For back health, add stretches in the other direction. Try these two after bicycling, gardening, cleaning floors, prolonged sitting, or any activity where you lean forward for prolonged periods:

1. Stand up with your hands on your behind. Lean back into an arch.
2. Another variation is to lie facedown. Slowly, gently press up into an arch, keeping your stomach flat on the floor or bed. Go only to the point where you feel stretch, not pain.

Figure 21.14. Take frequent breaks from sitting or working to stretch your back and neck.

Neck Stretches

1. For healthy neck range of motion, don't roll your head, just align your ears over your shoulders and look down, look up, look left, look right, and tip each ear to each shoulder. The bones of the neck were not made to roll around each other, a motion called circumduction. Excessive rolling is just wear and tear, and can be uncomfortable for the people with neck complaints.
2. Commonly, neck pain from a forward head posture is along the top of each shoulder, down from your neck, and around your shoulder blades. A good stretch to relieve this is to put one hand behind you in the opposite pocket (or imaginary pocket). Keep your face straight forward, then gently tilt your head toward your hand.

Tips to Avoid Back and Neck Pain

- Stand and sit keeping the normal inward curve of your lower back.
- Use a lumbar roll when sitting. Get one for the car, and take one with you.
- Regularly stretch your hamstrings, hip flexors, back, and neck.

- Do back exercises that include extension. Ab exercises alone are only one side of the ring of support that you need.
- Do leg exercises that develop your thigh and behind muscles (quadriceps and gluteal muscles) for the shock absorption your back needs, and to have the leg strength to be able to lift with your legs, not your back.
- Any time you bend over, bend your knees.
- Use proper lifting technique. When lifting anything, get close, face the weight, feet apart, bend your knees. Keep your torso upright. Lift slowly. Keep the weight close to you.
- Stand up after every half hour or so of sitting and stretch your back in the other direction.

Treating Back and Neck Pain

Because most ordinary back or neck pain goes away by itself (although temporarily), much confusion results about what relieved it. If you tried a home remedy, however far-fetched, you think the remedy worked. For this reason, the market is flooded with snake-oil potions for back pain. Understandably, many back and neck pain sufferers will try anything.

Address the Cause

Many people take back pain remedies, then go right back to the standing, sitting, and lifting problems that gave them the trouble in the first place. Then they eventually get more back and neck pain. They don't understand it. They call it stress. They try chiropractors, acupuncture, prescription and over-the-counter medications, psychotherapy, and prayer. They do everything except change the postural habits that got them into the mess. Some wind up in surgery, and still their pain persists. They think they are cursed. Luckily it does not have to be that way. See your physician for a good diagnosis, and instructions on how to begin a good back exercise program to speed recovery and decrease your chance of it recurring.

People take back pain remedies, then go right back to the
bad habits that gave them back pain in the first place.
They don't understand when their pain returns, because
they thought they were "fixed." But they didn't fix
the cause.

Diagnosis

Get an accurate diagnosis from a physician specializing in orthopedics. The Greek word *gnosis* means "knowing" or "recognizing." *Dia-*
is a word element that, in this context, means "completely." It's crucial
to completely know. Getting rid of pain and the disability that goes
with it means treating the cause. Don't let any practitioner treat you
without knowing what's wrong first, particularly for severe pain.

First Aid

Even though accurate diagnosis is so important, immediate treatment for most back pain is similar. Reduce inflammation that causes
pain by using antiinflammatory medications and ice packs. Relax
muscular spasm with muscle-relaxing medications and stretches. Medications are meant to be used for only the first day or so. Muscle
relaxers are not appropriate for long-term use for most back pain.
The entire purpose is to knock out the spasm right away, then let
your body heal. If you have back muscles in spasm, the pain can be
crippling, but it can be a simple matter to get out the spasm. A trained
massage therapist, physical therapist, or osteopath can identify spasm,
and stretch it out with special release techniques. The relief is quick,
and seems to be miraculous, but it is often a simple matter. Muscles
are not supposed to be left in spasm or produce a long-term condition.
For more on muscle spasm, *see* Chapter 30 on leg cramps.

Identify the things you do that caused the problem. Don't just injure
your back, allow it to go into spasm and pain, and go to someone
to "fix" it. It is not a fix. Make easy modifications in your routine to
avoid the whole problem in the future. Then, as pain subsides, begin
a good back exercise program to increase your resistance to future
injury. Use ice after your workouts and at the end of every long day.
The old thinking of long bed rest for back pain has been found to
be counterproductive. It just further weakens and deconditions you.
You need activity and the right back exercises.

Pain can usually be tremendously decreased by the proper exercises that relieve the muscle spasm or disc herniation that is causing the pain. Recent studies have emphasized how important it is to get early exercise after back injury, and how damaging total bed rest can be.

What About Shots?

Maybe you knew someone who had terrible back pain, got a shot, and was immediately fine. These shots are usually a special antiinflammatory, delivered right into the swollen, inflamed area. This is an alternative to taking antiinflammatories by mouth. Antiinflammatories reduce the space-occupying swelling and pain. Two important cautions are that corticosteroid injections temporarily stop the healing process and also make the area temporarily weak and susceptible to tearing. You must be careful to take it easy after these shots, to do no further harm to the area.

Surgery Rarely Needed

Surgery for disc protrusions, or herniations, is rarely necessary. This happy discovery was made when disc patients were referred to physical therapy for back exercises to condition them for the physical stress of surgery. By surgery time, most of the people didn't need any. Problems from surgery to remove a disc are that your bones need your discs for cushioning and to keep from grinding bone directly on bone. Without your discs, you are subject to early wear and tear, possibly predisposing you to early arthritis. That is why surgeons try to leave as much of the disc as possible when doing disc surgery.

Spinal fusion, which is surgery to fuse one vertebra to the next, is the extreme, last resort. The area no longer moves at all. This means that the vertebrae and discs above and below the fused sites must move more, for you to have even close to the function you had before your surgery. That means much more wear and tear on those sections than they were designed for. A problem with spinal fusion is when the person must return to have the next segments fused too, when they wear out from the trauma of working overtime next to a fused segment.

Most herniations, and their associated inflammation, will heal, shrink, and go back into place—if you let them, and that big "if" is up to you. Watch your posture while sitting and standing. When you sit, use a lumbar roll. See your physician for a prescription for back exercises that are right for you. Extension exercises usually bring good results to reduce pain, slowly allow the disc to return into place, and strengthen muscles to keep your posture healthy for your back. These exercises are easy for you to do yourself at home after a bit of instruction.

What's the most effective treatment for back or neck pain?
Not drugs, not surgery. Just simple exercises.

When You Wake Up

Disc pain is usually worst upon waking in the morning because your discs customarily swell a bit overnight. For injured discs, this normal swelling increases the pain. The thing you don't want to do when you awake is to immediately sit at the edge of the bed in flexion. No one should do that, particularly not anyone with disc trouble. It puts outward pressure on discs when they are the most vulnerable. Instead, turn facedown and lie propped slightly on your elbows, in extension, for a few moments or so. Lying prone reduces pain and pressure. (But don't fall back to sleep.)

When you first wake up, turn facedown and lie propped
slightly on your elbows for a few moments, instead of
sitting. In most cases, it's better for your discs.

When you get out of bed, and anytime you get up from a lying-down position, roll to your side first, then push up with your arms, rather than "curling up" with a sit-up motion. Rolling to the side is a good back habit for everyone.

Make sure that when making beds in the morning that you do not lean over and lift. Bend your knees, keep your torso upright, and use the usual safe lifting mechanics.

Practice "Safe Necks"

This section only touched on the basics of back and neck care. There are other conditions that contribute their share of back misery.

Figure 21.15. This stretch takes the tightness out of your neck and shoulders. Tip your ear toward your shoulder, keeping your face looking forward, not down. It only takes a moment to do this one. Try it often.

But the basics of safe back and neck habits apply to most back pain. Preventing back and neck pain is easier than treating it. Practice "Safe Necks" to keep your back and neck healthy and pain free.

Resources for More Information

AMERICAN PHYSICAL THERAPY ASSOCIATION
1111 N. Fairfax Street
Alexandria, Virginia 22314-1488
(800) 999-APTA
(703) 684-2782
fax (703) 684-7343
Booklets, referrals to local physical therapists, and on-line computer resources.

KRAMES COMMUNICATIONS
1100 Grundy Lane
San Bruno, CA 94066-9821
(800) 333-3032
fax (415) 742-9265
Many helpful, inexpensive, short booklets, including "Back Owners Manual" and "Neck Basics."

AMERICAN PODIATRIC MEDICAL ASSOCIATION
9312 Old Georgetown Road
Bethesda, MD 20814
(301) 571-9200

22

Calcium, Protein, Space Flight, Exercise, and Your Bones—A Detective Story

Current recommendations for the prevention of osteopo-rosis may actually be detrimental to health.

—J. Strain, researcher at the Biomedical Sciences Research Centre, University of Ulster, in *Med. Hypotheses,* 1988 Dec; 27(4): pp333-8.

Join me on an international detective story. The beginning is decep-tively simple. Your bones need calcium; milk has calcium. Then questions begin creeping in. Why do some American vegetarians have a lower incidence of osteoporosis than the general population? Why do some groups of Japanese, whose calcium intake is historically low, develop osteoporosis, while others don't? Why do African Bantu women, who eat relatively little calcium, have low rates of osteoporo-sis? Why doesn't the very-high-calcium diet of Eskimos prevent their suffering the highest rate of osteoporosis in the world? Why do astro-nauts lose bone in space no matter what they eat?

The detective story opens with four separate studies. Researchers at the Mayo Clinic found no correlation between calcium intake and age-related bone loss after bone finishes forming in early adulthood. Then at Tufts University, researchers concluded that calcium had no effect on preventing bone loss in the first five years or so after meno-pause. From Cornell came a study in 1989 reporting: "It was not clear that increased calcium intake has a significant impact on osteoporosis or other chronic diseases that have been linked to calcium nutriture." More work published in the *Journal of the American Medical Woman's*

Association concluded that calcium intake alone will "neither guarantee optimal bone growth nor protect against bone loss if other critical factors are missing."

The search for these critical factors begins with a trip back in time and the realization that calcium can be not only excreted from your body before it has any chance of connecting with your bones, but driven from existing bone.

Your Changing Bones

Your bones are alive. They continuously break down and rebuild. Throughout your life, you make new bone cells, and breakdown and assimilate old ones. That recycling process is your body doing its normal business of cell maintenance. You exchange about 3–5% of your bone cells every year this way. All is well as long as you replace at least as much as you lose, much like money in your bank account. As you age, you do less bone making, and more bone losing. That isn't bad by itself—it depends how much bone you start out with, and how much you lose. The good news is that these are things you can control, to a certain extent.

What Is Osteoporosis?

With osteoporosis, you lose too much bone, leaving spaces in your bones, making them porous and fragile. *Osteo-* is a Greek word element meaning "bone." *Porosis* means "porous." Osteoporosis is a serious degenerative bone disorder. Because bone loss is completely painless until you break a bone, you probably won't know that bone loss is happening in your body. Fractures then easily occur, from little or no noticeable cause. Healing time is long, sometimes never occurring. It is often too late at that point to reverse the process.

The Toll of Osteoporosis

Osteoporosis takes a heavy toll:

- Osteoporosis affects 15 to 20 million middle-aged and older people.
- Osteoporosis-induced hip and spine fractures are a major cause

of illness and death among older women and, as they live longer, among men as well.

- An estimated 1.5 million osteoporotic fractures occur in the United States yearly.
- One woman in three over the age of 65 will suffer fractures of the spine, and from 10–15% of all white women will fracture their hip.
- Hip fractures are fatal within one year in up to about 20% of the cases.
- Half of those surviving a hip or spine fracture never walk unaided again, leaving about a quarter of the elderly female population of the United States disabled by severe osteoporosis. These risks exceed a woman's risk of developing endometrial cancer or breast cancer.
- Occurrence in women is higher than in men; nevertheless, osteoporosis in men is a substantial problem in medicine and society.

Why Young People Need to Know About Bone Health

Osteoporosis is not something that just happens to old people; it begins in youth. Your bone density in later years depends on what you are doing right now. Risk factors during youth can reduce the bone density of a twenty- or thirty-year-old to the equivalent of someone in their seventies.

Until your midthirties your bones are in an active growth phase that will determine your peak amount of bone. Building high peak bone mass in youth is like saving more money in the bank now for retirement later. It allows you to lose bone later in life through normal processes, without falling to dangerously low amounts, as you make "withdrawals." After a variable plateau period up to around age 40, bone loss begins silently, varying greatly from your genetically determined potential, depending on your food and exercise habits.

Like heart disease, bone loss is a gradual process. The time to actively direct its course is now, to prevent it from becoming serious later. Once bone loss becomes serious, it is not reversible. By the time osteoporosis is usually diagnosed, from 50% to 75% of the bone mass may be gone from your skeleton.

Developing the most bone mass you can by the time your
skeleton matures in adulthood may be the best
protection against bone loss and fractures later on. It may
be that low peak bone mass, rather than greater than
average bone loss, causes osteoporosis.

Where Does Osteoporosis Affect You?

Three sites are most at risk for osteoporosis:

1. Wrist.
2. Upper back.
3. Upper leg bone where it joins your hip. This upper leg bone is
   what usually breaks when you hear of someone "breaking their
   hip" due to osteoporosis.

When bone thins too much in the upper back bones, they slowly
begin to crush. Because of many forces on these bones, the front of
each crushes more than the back, giving a wedge shape to each
bone. Wedge fractures create the classic humped-back or "Dowager's
Hump," with height losses up to five inches. The Hunchback of Notre
Dame probably had osteoporosis.

Falls may fracture a wrist that would not have otherwise broken.
A broken wrist may be a warning sign of osteoporosis impending in
the hip or back. Tooth loss is another early warning sign. So much
bone is lost from the jaw that teeth loosen, then are lost.

Why Are These Particular Sites at Risk?

About 1% of your skeletal calcium is readily available to supply
your daily body processes. This pool is stored mostly in your spine
bones called vertebrae, and the ends of your long bones in a spongy
supportive mesh called trabecular bone (tra-BECK-you-lar). When
your body needs calcium, it takes it first from these stockpiles. The

Figure 22.1. The main sites of bone loss with aging in both men and women are your upper back, wrist, and hip. The time to prevent problems later is now.

result is fractures of the wrist and vertebrae. These fractures occur mainly in women, because of decreased estrogen around menopause. Elderly men also may suffer from vertebral crush fractures.

In men and women over 75, both trabecular and cortical bone are lost. The dense surface of your bones is called cortical bone. Long bones like those in your arms and legs are mostly cortical bone. Loss of too much cortical bone causes hip fractures. These fractures occur easily, even from normal stresses, because of the weakened bone structure.

Factors Affecting Risk

It is unfortunately common to believe that osteoporosis prevention is simply a matter of drinking milk. There are many factors in osteoporosis, not all of which are completely understood. There are at least four major determinants of how much bone mass you can achieve in your younger years, how much you later lose, and consequently, of fracture risk: genetics, nutrition, hormonal factors, and how much you exercise.

Genetics

Differences in bone density exist among ethnic and racial groups. Bone mass diminishes with age in all ethnic populations; however, osteoporosis most often affects Caucasians. The bones of white people are typically less dense than those of African-Americans, Hispanics, and Asians at all age groups. There also may be inherited tendencies to osteoporosis among families. Bone density in healthy mother-daughter pairs correlates significantly. Daughters of women with osteoporosis have lower bone density in similar sites as their mothers. Peak bone size, mass, and density may be influenced by fathers as well. These tendencies can be countered with practices to protect bone density, described later in this section.

Nutrition

The role of high calcium intake in adulthood is not really clear. You not only need to get enough calcium; you need to avoid too much of things that cause you to lose calcium from your bones, and interfere with calcium absorption. Of the major determinants of risk of osteoporosis, nutrition is one of the easiest to take charge of in your life.

Protein. A succession of well-controlled studies published since 1920 chronicle increased urinary calcium loss with increased meat in the diet. In 1988, a published study by the Center in Mineral Metabolism and Clinical Research in Texas concluded that urinary calcium excretion due to the animal protein of milk raised the risk of osteoporosis. Studies find that animal protein increased calcium loss even with high calcium intake, and when the animal versus vegetable protein diet is constant with respect to sodium, potassium, calcium, phosphorus, magnesium, and total protein. This is explained by the high sulfur content of animal protein compared to vegetable protein. Sulfur elevates metabolic acid production leading to chronic bone calcium loss, and reduced calcium reabsorption.

One study found that by age 80, 1,600 women on a lacto-ovo vegetarian diet for at least 20 years had lost only 18% bone mineral compared to closely paired omnivore women who lost 35%. The effect of too much animal protein to increase urinary calcium loss and decrease bone density is also conjectured to raise risk of another disease of bone loss—tooth loss from gum bone ridge resorption. The less animal protein, the less the loss.

Copper. A 1988 study from the University of Ulster implicated mild dietary copper deficiency in osteoporosis in both humans and animals. Medical literature states copper is abundant in normal diets but doesn't take into consideration that there are common barriers to copper utilization. The lactose in dairy products may interfere with copper metabolism. High sugar intake increases urinary excretion of both calcium and copper.

Vitamin D. Availability of Vitamin D, required for calcium absorption in the small intestine, dwindles with aging: the kidney reduces Vitamin D synthesis, people reduce outdoor sun exposure, and the function or number of Vitamin D–binding receptors in your intestine declines.

Caffeine. Caffeine may increase urinary excretion of calcium, but relation to risk is uncertain.

Alcohol. Osteoporosis is more common in alcoholics than in nonalcoholics of the same age. Alcohol is directly toxic to bone cells. Alcoholism contributes to bone loss through poor nutrition, liver disease, malabsorption of calcium and Vitamin D, and abnormal parathyroid gland function.

Smoking. Smoking, like alcohol, seems to be directly toxic to bone cells. Cigarette smoking also interferes with calcium absorption and estrogen, and is associated with earlier menopause and bone loss than in nonsmokers.

Calcium. The issue of calcium requirement provokes all kinds of debate. Many factors affect calcium absorption and excretion, making it difficult to pin down just how much calcium you need. In the 1960s and 1970s, major textbooks of medicine did not consider calcium important in osteoporosis development or prevention, or only considered calcium malabsorption disorders. In the 1980s, a calcium mania swept the public. Although much is still unknown, it is pretty well established that calcium intake influences bone mass formation until adulthood. In this way, calcium reduces subsequent osteoporosis risk since someone with high bone mass at age 30 may lose bone through normal aging, yet have sufficient bone remaining at 75.

However, studies seem to show that calcium alone does not guarantee optimal bone growth in youth. Neither will it prevent bone loss with age in men, with estrogen-withdrawal in women, or with immobilization as in a cast or with bed rest, or with amenorrhea (ay-men-or-REE-ah), which is absence of the menstrual cycle. It is also not even a sure bet if increased dietary calcium affects bone density once you reach adulthood. There are just too many other variables. You need to remember all of them in order to have healthy bones, not just eat calcium.

Just drinking your milk or taking calcium pills will not stop osteoporosis. Bone density depends on many other things, one big factor is how much exercise you get.

Other Nutritional Factors. Obviously, many nutritional factors are involved in the health of any body system. Many other vitamins and minerals, not discussed here, play small and interacting parts in your continually changing bones. The purpose here was to identify the major players and give an overview of the processes.

Hormonal Factors

Several hormones influence bone density and risk of osteoporosis in both women and men.

Menopause and Amenorrhea. One effect of the hormone estrogen is that it increases calcium retention in bone. Estrogen level is a strong predictor of bone mass over time. Sharply reduced estrogen states occur with amenorrhea, and with natural and surgical menopause. Surgical menopause involves removal of the ovaries, or oophorectomy (oo-for-EK-tuh-mee). Menopausal women lose high amounts of bone regardless of calcium intake. The bones previously relied heavily on the presence of estrogen. During the first menopausal years, withdrawal of the body's estrogen production is a major change. It takes time to adjust to the loss. But by then, much loss has taken place.

Many things may cause menstrual irregularities, or loss of the menstrual cycle entirely (amenorrhea) in premenopausal women. It is popular to blame vigorous exercise, with some authorities going as far as stating that athletes who experience amenorrhea should be banned from further training. But exercise alone does not seem to be sufficient to cause amenorrhea. Decreased body fat and insufficient nutrition are also involved. It seems to be an obvious and natural evolutionary feature that, if conditions are so harsh as to cause lack of food and constant, harsh travel, women should not be reproducing. Physical resources were better reserved until easier times.

For modern athletes, physical exercise is important to preserving bone mass. Stopping an amenorrheic athlete from exercise is counter-productive. Investigation into other contributing factors can allow the athlete to continue vigorous training, with all its benefits of health and well-being.

Reduced Hormone Levels in Men. Testosterone has many functions, including a part in regulating bone mass. The stress of extended periods of extreme exercise on the body seems to send a signal to the brain to decrease levels of two hormones which stimulate the testes to produce testosterone. As hormone levels go down, risks of various reproductive and bone density problems go up. Much attention in the literature is paid to the role of hormones, exercise, and bone density in women, but unfortunately little about the phenomenon in men.

Depo-Provera. The contraceptive Depo-Provera (medroxy-progesteroneacetate) reduces estrogen production. Women taking Depo-Provera often lose bone mass in the early years of use, and can have bone density values below normal values. Bone loss in the later years of Depo-Provera use usually levels off, until approaching the normal rate of age-related fall.

Endometriosis Treatment. Treatment with nafarelin for endometriosis increases bone loss. Adding norethisterone (NET) to nafarelin treatment seems to have a bone-sparing effect. Ask you physician if this pertains to you.

Steroid Antiinflammatories. Long-term corticosteroid (steroid hormone) treatment is given for several conditions including rheumatoid arthritis. Over years of use, steroid antiinflammatories can cause bone density loss and increase risk of fracturing for both men and women. Osteoporosis prevention is an important issue for anyone taking steroid antiinflammatories for long periods of time.

Anorexia Nervosa

Anorexia nervosa is a condition of abnormal loss of appetite and refusal to eat. It results in emaciation and malnutrition. Anorexia nervosa is a major risk factor for osteoporosis in both men and women for several reasons. The diet is severely calcium deficient, and the loss of muscle and total body weight decreases resistive forces on bones. Bones need a physical stimulus for maintaining thickness.

Unchecked, anorexia can lead to decreases in estrogen production, and loss of regular menstrual function, which is another risk factor for osteoporosis. Estrogen is a hormone needed to maintain bone density.

Exercise

Exercise is extremely important in osteoporosis prevention. The job of your bones is to support your body against the pull of gravity. Your bones develop more when there is more need for them to resist gravity. The physical stress of muscle pulling on bone during exercise stimulates bone to thicken and strengthen. By contrast, lack of mechanical stress from lack of exercise, prolonged immobility such as in a cast, during bed rest, or from paralysis, sedentary lifestyle, and weightlessness during space flight leads to bone loss regardless of how much calcium you eat. Bone loss from extended immobilization may become permanent after about six months of inactivity. Bed rest so effectively reduces bone density that it is used as a model for bone loss in the microgravity of space.

Animals that hibernate go without activity for long periods. Their bodies produce chemicals that prevent bone loss. Humans are strongly susceptible to bone loss from inactivity, and require resistive exercise to keep bones dense and strong. Like muscular atrophy from lack of exercise, the bone atrophy of osteoporosis is a "use it or lose it" disease. Sedentary lifestyle is a major risk factor. Without exercise, you lose calcium from your bones no matter how much calcium you eat.

Physical activity can increase bone mass in all age groups. Movement alone is not enough; there must be active muscular resistance. Weight-bearing activity, for example walking or jogging, increases bone density, primarily of the lower body. Weight-loading exercise, usually weight lifting, can increase bone density at all sites including the upper body. Like nutrition and unlike genetics, physical activity is a potentially controllable risk factor.

Your body weight is another important influence on bone density. After all, carrying around your body weight is exercise. Obesity increases bone density. Furthermore, higher-weight postmenopausal women often have higher estrogen levels, another protective factor. Very lightweight people reduce the weight load on hip and leg bones. Reduced bone density from low body weight is a problem for extremely thin and anorexic people. These people benefit by weight lifting exercise to help build muscle and bone.

What About Swimming?

Swimming is not a weight-bearing activity. It is a point of great interest to swimmers and scientists whether swimming can increase bone mass. Muscles still pull on bone to move you through the water, but is it less than during weight bearing? It seems to depend on how hard you work out. Recent studies report that tough swimming workouts give plenty of bone-building resistance. If the only exercise you get is a casual swim, it is wise to augment that with weight lifting and weight-bearing activities.

What About Scuba Diving?

Like swimming, scuba diving is not a weight-bearing sport, except when you are lugging all your gear around. Regularly lifting scuba gear is a good weight-loading activity for healthy backs. If you are able, carry your own tanks to get weight-lifting exercise. If your back is already osteoporotic, it may not be good to carry or wear your tank before you get into the water. The weight could further compress fragile vertebrae. In this case, don your tank in the water. Buoyancy underwater helps offset the weight of a tank. Check with your physician about diving safely if you have osteoporosis.

How Much Calcium Do You Need?

With so many interacting variables, your calcium need varies. You need more calcium if you lose calcium from smoking, drinking alcohol, and eating high amounts of animal protein. High intake of animal protein may cause calcium levels to become inadequate in situations where a tendency to low dietary calcium already exists. You may do well with less calcium if you exercise and reduce factors involved in calcium loss.

Although much is unknown, it is established that calcium intake influences bone mass until adulthood. In this way calcium reduces subsequent osteoporosis risk, since someone with high bone mass at age 30 may lose bone through normal aging yet have sufficient bone remaining at 75. It is not known if calcium intake over a certain minimum during adulthood influences bone density. Neal Barnard, M.D., President of the Physicians' Committee for Responsible Medicine (PCRM), reminds us that, "Excessive calcium intake does not fool hormones into building much more bone, any more than delivering an extra load of bricks will make a construction crew build a larger building." PCRM filed a complaint with the Federal Trade Commission against ads showing celebrity milk mustaches, stating that a few of them deceptively imply that just drinking milk will prevent bone loss.

Whether or not extra calcium will help, it is important to get enough calcium. In 1997, a panel of the Institute of Medicine, National Academy of Sciences, recommended a daily minimum RDA for calcium:

- 1300 mg/day for adolescents
- 1000 mg for adults 18 to 50
- 1200 mg over 50

Some authorities feel that most people do not get enough calcium. See your physician to determine your calcium needs.

Calcium Sources

What are good sources of calcium? Where do cows get theirs? You can't digest grass but dark green vegetables like spinach, collards, and kale are good sources of calcium. It used to be often stated that certain components of these plants, called phytate and oxalic acid, would depress calcium absorption, making them far less effective than dairy sources. However, calcium absorption from both low- and high-phytate soybeans was found to be close to that of milk, with absorption from low-phytate soybeans slightly higher than that of milk. Another recent study found interference by oxalic acid to be less than previously thought.

Broccoli has more calcium per calorie than any other food. Tofu has plenty, depending how it is processed. Seaweed is another good, yet frequently overlooked source. Fruit has calcium. So do almonds and sunflower seeds. Better yet, fruits, vegetables, nuts, and legumes have the element boron, which may participate in preventing osteoporosis. Milk has little boron. Meat and eggs have none. Because calcium absorption goes down with increased intake, spread out your daily dose into spaced intervals to increase absorption.

Can You Get Enough Calcium Without Dairy?

Although dairy products are the prevailing calcium source in many Western countries, they are not the only source, or even in some cases, the best source.

Dairy products do contain high amounts of calcium which are well absorbed. Still, there are problems with dairy products for many people:

- Dairy is one of the most potent causes of allergy.
- Dairy is a major source of fat and cholesterol.
- The capacity to break down the milk sugar galactose decreases with age. Galactose may be associated with cataracts and ovarian cancer.
- Dairy products contain lactose. Many people lose the ability to digest lactose after childhood, causing gas and pain.
- Lactose may interfere with copper metabolism. A mild deficiency of copper, common in Western diets, is related to the development of osteoporosis.
- The animal protein in dairy can increase urinary calcium loss.

It is not difficult to get adequate calcium without dairy products. Many non-Western people get more calcium than the average American, from nondairy sources. Peruvian Indians eat cereal mixed with powdered calcium carbonate rock. Contemporary hunter-gatherers have a high calcium intake, three times higher than the average middle-age American woman, without eating any dairy.

What About Calcium Supplements?

Calcium supplements are major sales items, even though major health organizations recommend getting calcium from food, not supplements. The U.S. Food and Drug Administration recommends check-

High-Calcium Foods

Source	Milligrams of Calcium (mg)
1 cup tofu processed with calcium sulfate	868
1 cup dulse seaweed	600
1 cup navy beans & 2 corn tortillas	370
1 cup milk	291
1 cup amaranth	280
1 cup kale	200
1 cup broccoli	180
1 cup soybeans	175
1 tablespoon blackstrap molasses	140
1 cup fortified orange juice	120
1 cup dried apricots	100

ing the labels of many kinds of bottled calcium pills, to avoid bone meal and dolomite sources because of their high content of lead and other toxic metals. Calcium carbonate is a good alternative.

Calcium absorption among the various supplement tablets is generally good, particularly between meals, except in people who underproduce stomach acid. For these people, taking calcium tablets with a meal benefits absorption. Since three times the dose is needed for some people to absorb the same amount of calcium, absorption fraction should be assessed by a physician before beginning a supplement regimen. Most, but not all supplements are easily absorbed. A common test is to put the calcium tablet in a glass of vinegar. If it dissolves within 30 minutes, it is more likely to be absorbed in your digestive tract than those that won't dissolve in the vinegar.

How to Reduce Your Risk of Osteoporosis

You can control several things to reduce your risk:

- Get regular exercise. An effective bone-building exercise is lifting weights. Also important is resisting your own body weight during weight-bearing exercise like walking, dancing, running, skating, and skiing.

- Get adequate calcium from a variety of sources, and spread your intake throughout the day.
- Quit smoking.
- Drink less alcohol.
- Avoid high-meat diets.
- Alcoholics should be screened periodically for Vitamin D deficiency and bone loss, and get Vitamin D supplements when either is detected.
- Various drug treatments effectively combat osteoporosis after menopause. Estrogen replacement is the best known. Until recently, estrogen replacement was often considered the only way to maintain bone mass in the first five years after menopause. Estrogen replacement also reduces cholesterol, and cuts risk of heart attack by approximately 50% compared to women without replacement. Estrogen replacement may increase the risk of uterine or breast cancer in susceptible women, but since many more women die of heart attack than hip fracture or cancer, the benefits of estrogen can outweigh the smaller risk of cancer for those not already at risk. Estrogen replacement is also questionable for women at risk for stroke. More nonhormonal drugs are becoming available that work to prevent and treat osteoporosis without the cancer risk, but also without the cardiovascular benefits. New designer estrogens have bone- and heart-saving benefits without the risks of breast and uterine cancers sometimes associated with estrogen replacement. Women with risk factors for osteoporosis and a history or risk of stroke, heart disease, or any cancer should weigh the relative benefits and risks of the various medications with their physician.

OSTEOPOROSIS RISK REDUCTION

Reduce	Increase	Consider
Inactivity and sedentary lifestyle	Physical activity, including weight-bearing activity	Osteoporosis prevention medications after menopause
Animal protein	Vegetable protein	Bone density evaluation
Alcohol	Weight lifting	Nutritional assessment
Smoking	Vegetable-based calcium	Reducing caffeine, salt

Important Answers

So the detective story, while not solved, revealed crucial clues. Populations in Japan whose low protein intake comes primarily from plant sources have normal bone growth and low rates of age-related osteoporosis even with calcium intakes half that recommended in the United States. In their genetic relatives eating a modern diet, high salt and protein intake aggravates calcium deficiency in old age. African Bantu women eat less than half the currently recommended calcium, and have low rates of osteoporosis. They eat predominantly plant protein. Their genetic relatives living in the United States eating the Western diet of high animal protein suffer rates of osteoporosis and fractures similar to those of other North Americans. Eskimos have a high-calcium diet—nearly twice the recommended amount—and are physically active, yet suffer the world's highest rate of osteoporosis, which scientists relate to their high animal protein diet.

Calcium is not the whole story in bone health. Getting enough calcium is crucial, but without other critical factors, it is not a cure-all. Osteoporosis affects both men and women. Attaining high peak bone density when younger reduces the chance of lowering bone mass to unhealthy levels in later life.

Factors affecting your risk:

- How much exercise you get.
- Your total nutritional picture.
- Your heredity.
- Your hormonal status.

Reducing calcium loss may be as important as getting enough. Factors that increase your calcium loss:

- Lack of exercise.
- Smoking.
- High alcohol intake.
- High-protein diet.

To build bone and reduce bone loss:

- Increase physical activity.
- Get adequate nutrition.
- Estrogen replacement or other bone building medications after menopause (determined by your physician).

The most important message is not to wait until later. Preventing osteoporosis later depends on what you are doing right now.

Resources for More Information

PHYSICIANS FOR RESPONSIBLE MEDICINE
P.O. Box 6322
Washington, DC 20015
(202) 686-2210

NATIONAL OSTEOPOROSIS FOUNDATION
2100 M Street N.W., Suite 602
Washington, DC 20037
(202) 223-2226

23

Body Fat—It's Not All Bad

Am I fat? I've fallen down and not even known it.

—Pat McCormick

Some people worry when they don't fit into their tightest suit. Others don't worry until they can't fit into the car. A quick look around reveals that being a little plump seems to be the norm. Is that all bad?

When Does Fat Help You?

You could not live without a certain amount of body fat. Fat is a necessary part of every cell in your body. Your nerves could not conduct signals rapidly enough for you to function without their fatty wrapping.

Body fat keeps you warm in the cold. Without a certain minimum of body fat, you lose your reproductive ability.

Fat pads the discomfort of sitting and standing, and carrying shoulder bags and backpacks, and blows to your internal organs. High body weight, whether from fat or lean, provides the loading your bones need to stay dense and strong. Obese people have low rates of osteoporosis.

Success in different sports depends on characteristic body sizes and compositions. Football linemen almost always have more than an average amount of fat compared to other athletes. Fat weight is an advantage to linemen for the added mass and padding for blocking ability. Increased muscle mass accompanies the extra fat weight to carry the whole package around.

Sumo wrestling is another sport where extra fat weight helps. Linemen and sumos don't have to run around much. It's not a big disadvantage to carry extra weight. Other sports where the players have more fat than average for athletes are baseball, discus throwing, ice hockey, and swimming.

Figure 23.1. High body fat benefits some activities.

Study after study confirms a direct relation between body fat and keeping warm in the cold—helpful in sports like swimming, ice hockey, ice fishing, skiing, and other cold weather activities. You don't have to be obese for thermal benefits. Any amount of fat adds insulation.

Because of the extra work of carrying around extra fat, a heavy person generally develops extra muscle mass. Heavy people not only have more pounds of fat than lighter people but more pounds of muscle. Extra muscle comes in handy in work like lifting things, as well as keeping warm in the cold. Consider the extra fat as a built-in daily weight-lifting regime.

Fat increases buoyancy, adding safety and comfort to swimming. A little fat on your legs lets you float more horizontally, which is a better body position for moving efficiently through the water for scuba diving and swimming. Skinny legs often tend to sink, ruining streamline.

When Does Fat Hinder You?

Extra fat weight is a burden to carry across distance or against gravity. Extra fat weight is more work to carry around. The high-calorie cost of transporting extra weight makes low body fat advantageous to gymnastics, climbing, and any sport where you have to run or run around. World-class distance runners almost always have extremely low body fat. Runners and gymnasts, along with boxers and wrestlers, often adopt unhealthy dietary restrictions trying to keep their weight low enough to help them in their chosen sport.

The same fat that keeps you warm in the cold makes you warm in hot weather, too. One predisposing factor to overheating is being large, round, and fat.

Having enough fat for health, comfort, and optimal performance in your sport is important. The next chapter describes the problems of too much of a good thing.

BODY FAT OF ATHLETES IN DIFFERENT SPORTS

Higher-Fat Athletes	Lower-Fat Athletes
Swimmers	Distance runners
Football linemen	Gymnasts
Sumos	Acrobats
Baseball players	Climbers
Ice hockey players	Boxers
Water polo players	Wrestlers

24

Problems of Being Overweight

Those who think they have no time for bodily exercise
will sooner or later have to find time for illness.

—Edward Stanley

Fat has benefits, as discussed in the previous chapter. Too much fat has drawbacks, among them, increased risk of orthopedic problems, heart attack, stroke, diabetes, certain cancers, gastrointestinal problems, and even a higher incidence of snoring.

It is estimated that slightly over 40% of American men are overweight compared to just under 30% of American women. Paradoxically, up to one-half of American women but only one-fourth of American men are estimated to be on a weight-reduction program at any point in time. This seems to be the case, even though women may be less active in organized exercise activities and sports. They just may be more weight conscious. The disparity often results in a phenomenon called "The Flintstones," where couples consist of an overweight man and a slimmer woman.

Heavy Consequences

More Work

It takes extra energy, work, and calories to carry extra fat around, depending on the work load. This is why a heavy man may work harder and closer to his maximum than a lighter man or woman to do physical activity that moves his body against gravity—for example, walking, running, climbing a hill, ascending stairs, and dancing. This is often the case even if the lighter person has a lesser physical capacity.

On one hand, you could say that extra work is free exercise and be happy about it. For heavy people in good physical shape, the extra work falls within their comfort range. For those in so-so to poor shape, this work can be beyond the capacity of the out-of-shape heart to supply itself and the body with oxygen, beyond the capacity of fat-narrowed blood vessels to conduct enough blood, or past the ability of the joints to chronically support the weight.

Illness and Injury

First, there's the obvious. Backaches, sore knees, achy feet—all more common for those who are greatly overweight. There's the old-hat stuff about heart disease, stroke, cancer, osteoarthritis, and gall bladder trouble all increasing with poundage. A large percentage of adult-onset diabetes cases in predisposed men are triggered by obesity. Adult-onset diabetes deteriorates blood vessels, sometimes ending in blindness and the loss of legs. Overweight is one of several factors combining to result in diverticulitis, a painful inflammation of the large intestinal wall. Overweight is a contributor in hernia, eventually affecting one out of eight men.

Snoring

Then there are the problems no one tells you about. High body fat is a key contributor to serious snoring and its more problematic relative, sleep apnea. Sleep apnea is a sleep disorder where the snorer stops breathing during sleep, sometimes hundreds of times per night. The large, heavy neck and throat of being overweight leads to upper airway obstruction. Bouts of oxygen starvation occur during sleep, and the person may frequently wake up gasping and snorting. Over time, lack of oxygen to the blood vessels results in fatty deposits in the blood vessels of the heart and brain. This is thought to be one of the mechanisms for the higher incidence of stroke and cardiac irregularities in people with this sleep disorder.

Other long-term, harmful effects from snoring-related sleep disorders are more subtle but equally dangerous—the repeated awakenings from the snoring and apnea result in chronic daytime sleepiness. This sleepiness is documented to greatly raise the risk of serious automobile accidents—by some estimates, up to seven times more accidents.

Sleep apnea is sometimes called the Pickwickian syndrome, after the "Fat Boy" in Dickens' *Pickwick Papers,* who was obese and sluggish in the daytime. In Greek mythology, Ondine (alternately spelled Undine) was a water sprite who cursed a poorly behaving man to thereafter breathe only voluntarily, not automatically. When he fell asleep, he stopped breathing and suffocated. For modern sufferers of Ondine's curse, losing weight is often the first line of medically prescribed treatment.

Death

A man just 20% overweight is twice as likely as a normal-weight man to die before age 50 from a weight-related disease. Just 20%. That's a man who should weigh close to 170 pounds (77 kilograms), but weighs over 200 pounds (91 kilograms).

Scary Stuff

Then there's the scary stuff. "Cognitive decline" was linked to circulatory disorders resulting from obesity in a Cornell Medical College study published in the February 1992 *Clinical Geriatric Medicine.* Data reported in the September 1992 issue of *Hypertension* indicate that men with long-term high blood pressure lost left brain tissue compared to men with normal blood pressure. A high percentage of high blood pressure cases are linked to being overweight, even without high salt intake. The researchers suspect the specific areas of brain tissue loss affect memory, language, and "finding your way around."

25

How to Tell How Much Fat You've Got

You know you're getting fat when you can pinch an inch on your forehead.

—John Mendoza

Many people carry more than a healthy amount of body fat. How do you know if you're one of them? There are many tests, some you can do yourself at home or the gym with simple equipment. Some require only minimal training. Others need sophisticated measurement machinery run by skilled operators and interpreters.

In general, for your own use, focus on the ideas, rather than the specific numbers. Reducing your fat weight helps to lessen your chance of the diseases and problems mentioned in Chapter 24, "Problems of Being Overweight," particularly if you are at risk for them anyway. But finding out what the tests are and how they are done is an interesting story.

Apples and Pears

Where you carry your fat is as important, or some say more so, than how much you have. The apple versus pear test requires only a mirror. Carrying fat primarily in the upper body and abdomen gives an apple shape to your figure. Lower body fat distributed on the hips and thighs makes a body more pear-shaped. Apple-shaped people seem to have a greater risk of obesity-related disease like heart disease, colon cancer, diverticulitis, diabetes, and high blood pressure than the pear-shaped. In short, beer bellies are more a health risk than thunder thighs.

Waist to Hip Ratio

The waist to hip ratio test further defines the apple vs. pear test. It just looks to see if your waist is big compared to your hips. You find this out by taking your waist and hip measurements, and dividing the waist by the hip measurement. Answers above 0.8 for women and 1.0 for men indicate a tendency toward the more problematic apple shape. For example, waist 37 inches, hip 36 inches (94 cm and 92 cm). The answer is 1.03, not good for anyone.

Insurance Tables

One way to predict health, according to insurance companies, is to check your weight against values in their insurance company tables that tell the ideal weight for your height. According to the height and weight tables of the Metropolitan Life Insurance Company, if you are more than 20% above their supposed ideal weight, you are considered obese. Exercise scientists recommend against relying on insurance tables, as there were problems in the procedures for developing them, and like other tests limited to height and weight, they ignore the fact that people have considerable variations in the amount of body fat for their height and weight.

Body Mass Index

The Body Mass Index (BMI) compares how heavy you are relative to your height. To calculate BMI divide your weight in kilograms by your height in meters squared. According to this test, if your BMI is over 25, you are fat. Above 30, you are considered obese. This test, like insurance tables, does not distinguish very muscular people from those overfat, and misses light, yet high-fat people.

For example, at 5'10" (1.78 meters), a weight above 174 pounds

(79 kg) is fat, above 209 pounds (95 kg) tips your BMI over 30. At 5'4" (1.63 m) your BMI passes 25 at weights above 146 pounds (66 kg) and 30 at weights above 175 pounds (80 kg).

Feet and Meters, Pounds and Kilos?

The United States still uses units of measurement historically based on royal anatomy and pottery; the foot, gallon, pound, etc. Most of the rest of the world uses the metric system, with comparable units of the meter, liter, and kilogram. How to convert one to the other?

Kilos to Pounds: 1 kilogram is about 2.2 pounds, so multiply the number of kilos by 2.2 to get pounds.
Pounds to Kilos: 1 pound is about 0.45 kilogram, so multiply the number of pounds by 0.45 to get kilograms.
Meters to Feet: 1 meter is about 3.3 feet, so multiply the number of meters by 3.3 to get feet.
Feet to Meters: 1 foot is about 0.3 meters, so multiply the number of feet by 0.3 to get meters.

Somatotyping

Height and weight tests do not account for your musculature and body dimensions. Somatotyping is a method of classifying your body according to three characteristics—thinness, fatness, and muscularity. Thinness is called ectomorphy. Fatness is called endomorphy. Muscularity is called mesomorphy. Each type has specific characteristics of limb and body dimensions, with varying proportions of fat, bone, and muscle.

No one is only one somatotype. Everyone is a mixture of the three types in differing amounts. Some people predominate in one type, giving them the long, linear and delicate appearance of the ectomorph; the round, soft, and short-necked look of the endomorph; or the hard, square, and rugged muscled body of the mesomorph. In football many players score high in both mesomorphy and endomorphy. Swimmers are usually ecto-mesomorphs. Gymnasts are usually ecto-meso-morphs. Sprint runners score higher in mesomorphy than distance runners. Coaches use somatotyping to identify those who would excel in different sports.

Casual somatotyping is done by the eyeball technique. Complete somatotyping requires trained analysis, photographs, or close inspection of naked subjects in three planes, caliper skinfold measurements, reference tables, and equations.

Anthropometrics

As part of somatotyping, or as a separate assessment, the size of the body's frame is determined with calculations using measurements of bone lengths and widths. Knowing frame size helps determine optimum weight. One test, the Heath-Carter, measures elbow width, knee width, biceps circumference, and calf circumference. Another anthropometric test, the Skeletal Frame Technique, measures widths of the shoulder and hip. The Tipton technique computes the minimum healthy weight for a given frame based on width and depth of the chest, and width of the ankle, wrist, and hip at two sites.

Index Tests

The Ponderal Index is your height divided by the cube root of your weight. Ponderal Index is used to determine degree of endomorphy. The Quetelet Index is another simple index of general body proportion. The Circumference Test is nothing more than the familiar tape measure around the waist, hip, chest, leg, arm, or whatever.

The Jiggle Test

Jump in the air. When you land, see how long it takes for all your parts to stop jiggling. Higher times indicate higher fat amounts.

Are You Fat?

Apples and Pears. Is your body apple-shaped with fat primarily in the upper body and abdomen, or pear-shaped with fat mostly on the hips and thighs? Those with the apple shape tend toward obesity-linked disease.

Waist-to-Hip Ratio. Take your waist and hip measurements. Divide your waist measurement by your hip measurement. Stay below 0.8 (women) and 1.0 (men).

Insurance Tables. Compare your weight against values in tables. More than 20% over this weight range indicates that you are considered obese.

Body Mass Index. The Body Mass Index (BMI) measures how heavy you are compared to your height. Divide your weight in kilograms by your height in meters squared. If your BMI is above 25, you are considered fat. If over 30, you are considered obese.

Somatotyping. Somatotyping classifies your body according to three characteristics—thinness or ectomorphy, fatness or endomorphy, and muscularity or mesomorphy.

Anthropometrics. Measuring bone lengths and widths at specific joints tells the size of your body's frame—small, medium, or large, which helps determine optimum weight.

The Jiggle Test. Jump in the air. When you land, see how long it takes for all your parts to stop jiggling. Higher times indicate higher fat amounts.

Measuring Percentage Body Fat

The different assessments talked about so far give an indirect estimation of your fat distribution. If you want to find out how much fat is actually attached to your body, you need body composition tests. These tests estimate what percentage of your total weight is just fat.

Why Measure Percentage Body Fat?

A slender-looking person of normal weight can have a high amount of body fat. Another person weighing above average for their height may have heavy musculature and little body fat. The second person is above average weight, yet has low body fat. The first is normal weight and overfat, even though not seeming to be. The difference is in their amount of body fat relative to their total weight, or percent body fat.

What's "Average" Body Fat?

For comparison purposes, a healthy body fat is usually given as 10–15% for men and 15–25% for women. Percentages lower than that are considered thin. Higher figures are considered to be fat. Figures very much above those are considered to be very fat. As an interesting note, recent studies reveal the average American, male or female, is closer to 22% fat.

Body Fat Tests

The only way to directly find out the specific amount of body fat you have would be to cut your body apart and try to scoop out all the fat stores. Even this direct method would miss fat deep inside and scattered around internal organs. All the other body fat tests are estimates.

There are several methods for estimating your percentage of body fat. These tests are called body composition analysis. Accuracy of some tests is poor, others moderate to pretty accurate to within a few percent. Here are a few of the most common ones.

Calipers

Calipers measure the thickness of your folds of fat. This is also sometimes called the "pinch test." Calipers are a small, simple, and inexpensive instrument. There are several caliper tests that use up to ten sites on your body. Simple equations translate the sums of different sites into percent fat. Caliper measurement is painless unless the tester too enthusiastically grabs and squeezes. The error of measurement of testing percent fat with calipers can be large, up to about 3–7%, varying greatly with the experience of the tester, making it not a true measure but a gross estimation. Caliper testing is often misused, particularly in health clubs. If a first reading shows 25% fat, then weeks later after an exercise program the second reading is 22%, it does not necessarily mean the person lost 3% fat. The large error of measurement makes it impossible to tell. Not all calipers read the same either. It is like a bathroom scale that weighs you at 160 one time, at 170 the next, and 150 the third time when you haven't changed weight.

Hydrostatic Weighing

Hydrostatic weighing, also called underwater weighing, is currently the gold standard of body composition analysis techniques. It has the lowest percentage error of all current body composition tests. There are two main methods of underwater weighing, and several different equations. One underwater weighing method uses Archimedes' principle. Density is mass/volume. You know your mass, and find your volume with water displacement.

Another method obtains body volume by subtracting your weight in water from weight in air. You sit on a scale in a tank of water and exhale as fully as you can with your head under water. The rest of the air that is left in your lungs after you exhale maximally is called residual volume. Residual volume can either be directly determined before the underwater weighing, or estimated with population charts. Your body density is determined from equations of your weight underwater minus your residual volume. The final reading can be off if you are unwilling to exhale completely underwater and hold the exhale for as long as it takes for the tester to get a good measurement. Being gassy can affect your results.

Near Infrared Interactance (NIR)

NIR is a technique based on the absorption of light in your fat versus your lean mass. Generally, manufacturers haven't burdened themselves with input from scientists in developing it, and there is some feeling that the technology has a long way to go. Some units claiming to use infrared interactance don't use it, rendering the unit even less accurate.

Other Tests

Sophisticated body composition analysis includes bioelectric impedance, potassium ion determination, ultrasound, CAT scans, creatine absorption, proton absorptionmetry, and nuclear magnetic resonance imagery. These tests require expensive equipment, and need further validation to know just how good they are.

What to Do?

Once you know your body composition, what can you do about it if you don't like it? The next section explains what you can do about the shape you're in.

26

What to Do About the Shape You're In

It is a hard matter, my fellow citizens, to argue with the belly since it has no ears.

—Cato the Elder (Roman politician and general)

But argue with the belly we do. Constantly. Weight control is a multibillion-dollar industry of widgets, gimmicks, and programs, some legit, some less so.

Weight control also is usually a dismal failure. People trying to lose weight lose muscle, bone, water, electrolytes, but not an appreciable amount of fat. When they regain the weight, as most dieters do, they gain back fat. Plenty of people want to put on lean weight, but wind up putting on fat weight. The body is designed to survive. Fat helps that to a degree, so the body holds dearly to its fat. What if you don't like the idea of holding dearly to your fat? If you and your physician have determined you have more than enough of a good thing, what can you do about it? This section describes what to do to lose a little, what not to do, and why we even have body fat at all.

Why You Have Fat and Plants Don't

You don't often see a fat plant. With few exceptions like avocados, coconuts, and other nuts, plants don't store their energy in the form of fat. We do. Why is this?

Being fat is often equated with being heavy, ponderous, weighty.

Yet, fat is lightweight compared to protein and carbohydrate. The same volume of fat weighs less than muscle protein. One of fat's famous traits is being light enough to float.

Fat has twice the calories as the same quantity of carbohydrate or protein by weight. In that way, fat stores more energy than carbohydrate or muscle. This lightweight, energy-dense storage form is the reason animals use fat as a storage vehicle. If you have to carry your energy around with you, it makes sense to make it a lightweight package.

Plants are mellow. Plants don't go places often. Their storage medium does not require weight control. They store most of their energy as carbohydrate. The extra weight is not a metabolic burden. Plants are heavy for their size. Ask any tree.

Why are avocados and coconuts exceptions? Because they, like other seeds and nuts, are the portion of plants that must move. They travel to new locations to germinate. They typically store fat to make their energy suitcases lighter.

Animals store little energy in the form of carbohydrate. Meat has, for all practical purposes, no carbohydrate. This is true even though your muscles stock a carbohydrate called glycogen that you use in short bouts of exercise. Your carbohydrate cache is so small that your muscle, and the muscles you eat if you are a meat eater, is partly protein, a good deal of fat (even in lean cuts), but no carbohydrate that makes any difference nutritionally.

Plants store their energy as carbohydrate, which is heavier than the same volume of fat. The extra weight is not a burden since plants don't travel. Avocados and coconuts are exceptions because they, like other seeds and nuts, are the portion of plants that move to new locations to germinate.
Animals carry their energy around with them so it makes sense to carry it in a lightweight package—fat.

Why You Get Fat

So, humans have fat, but why so much in some cases? There are studies that show that fat people often don't eat a whole lot more calories than thinner people do. The difference is mainly in the amount of exercise they get and what kind of food they eat.

It's easy to be sedentary, particularly in a lifestyle geared around the automobile and television. Our daily life is not usually active. Weekend warriors rarely exercise enough for it to count as regular exercise. It's easy to pack on a few pounds if you don't routinely exercise in other ways.

Being fat usually results from too little exercise.

How to Lose Fat: What Not to Do

People flock to outrageous weight loss regimes, programs, gizmos, and outright hoaxes. Why are starvation, dehydration, stomach stapling, unhealthy fad diets, vibrating machines, and amphetamines considered acceptable, while exercise is avoided as extreme? Avoid unhealthy gimmicks in favor of a healthy lifestyle. Healthy exercising is detailed in Part I of this book.

Don't Fad Diet

Fad diets restrict your nutrition, are usually not healthy, and don't keep the weight off in the long run. Severe calorie restriction by itself is rarely successful and hard to sustain. Don't forget that many so-called diets are just gimmicks. Just because something is called a diet doesn't mean it is a weight-loss diet. After all, anything you eat is your diet—it could be all ice cream and cardboard boxes.

Don't Restrict Water

Water is not fat. Losing water weight has no effect on fat loss. You need water to be healthy. Don't restrict water in hopes of losing water weight. Dehydration is unhealthy in general for your body, lowers your exercise capacity, and your ability to thermoregulate. For those who eat when they're not hungry, a glass of water is a good substitute.

Don't Lose Weight Quickly

Quick weight loss usually returns just as quickly. It's also tough on your heart. Avoid rapid weight loss unless your physician has determined that the benefits outweigh the risks. The more slowly you lose weight, the more likely it is to stay off.

Don't Believe Claims of Spot Reducing

Spot reducing is a myth. The idea of spot reducing is to lose fat from a specified area by repetitive movement of that area. If that were true, then the people selling spot-reducing devices and overeaters would have thin mouths from all their talking, and bicycle riders would have skinny legs. If you want to lose fat, then do aerobic exercise like walking, running, biking, cross-country skiing, rowing, and swimming.

Remember Error of Measurement

Don't believe health club personnel that measure your body fat with calipers at intervals and state that you have lost 2% fat, or 5% fat, or whatever percent since starting their program. The error of body fat measurement inherent in caliper testing is too high to compare specific percents over time. Trust the fit of your clothing. *See* Chapter 25, "How to Tell How Much Fat You've Got," for more about fat measurement.

Don't Hate Yourself

Accept yourself if you have a little more to adore. If you are meant to be big, appreciate the advantages. Be sure to exercise and trim food fat for health. Anorexia and starvation are passé. Being big isn't for everyone, but neither is being too thin. There's no reason you can't be big-boned, large, healthy, and happy too.

How to Lose Fat—What Not to Do

- Avoid gimmicks.
- Don't fad diet, and don't eat high-sugar, high-calorie foods just because they are "fat-free."

- Don't restrict water.
- Don't lose weight too quickly.
- Don't believe claims of spot reducing. To lose fat, do aerobic activities like walking, dancing, skating, or biking.
- Don't hate yourself.

How to Lose Fat: What to Do

There are plenty of easy, even fun ways to lose fat. Here are a few.

Give Peas a Chance

Remember, animals have fat and plants generally don't. Eat more plants. Meat, even lean cuts, often have more than the maximum amount of fat recommended by the American Heart Association. Vegetables and grains are a good source of carbohydrate that fuels your body. Plants are a good source of protein, but unlike meat, have no cholesterol and little fat. It used to be thought that plant protein was not as good as meat protein. In the modern diet there is little chance of not getting enough of the different kinds of protein you need from vegetable sources. There is no need to carefully combine plant proteins, as once thought. Your body does that for you automatically, as you eat over the days.

Eat Low Fat

So-called sensible eating means not starving yourself. Just exchange a few bad food preferences for healthier ones. Find low-fat substitutes for habitual high-fat snacks. Chapter 15, "Calculating Food Fat," explains how to tell how much fat is in the foods you eat, and lists fat contents of common foods. Develop some fun, healthful, new food preferences.

Not all calories are the same. When you eat one hundred calories of carbohydrate, your body burns 25 calories just to digest the carbohydrate. When you eat one humdred

calories of fat, your body burns just three calories to
process it.

Reclaim Built-in Exercise

Many activities of daily living are built-in exercise. Devices like garage door openers greatly benefit those with health problems that would be aggravated by opening the heavy door. For others, opening the door twice a day, so many days per week, would give you extra muscle and lose you a few pounds of fat per year. You can find many other examples throughout your day like swapping walking for driving, steps for elevators, push mowers for power mowers, carrying your own packages and golf clubs rather that using a cart— you get the idea. Exercising in a gym is really only a substitute for having an active lifestyle. Some people prefer to drive to a health club and take the elevator to their exercise class. Others hate the gym, and are thrilled to find they can avoid it by having a fun, active life.

Read About Fitness

Get educated. Read this book. Read all you can.

See Your Physician

See your physician to determine your general state of health and percent body fat. Choose a physician skilled in this area.

Exercise

Exercise is the key to losing excess body fat. Exercise doesn't only mean going to the gym. Find a few regular activities that you enjoy, that fit your lifestyle, and that you can build into your ordinary day without it being a chore.

Exercise

Find a few regular activities that you enjoy, that fit your lifestyle, and that you can build into your ordinary day without it being a chore.

Lift Weights

Weight lifting is important to fitness. Lifting weights alters your body composition toward the lean, burns calories, and helps you get fit and have more fun through an active life. *See* Chapter 3, "Improving Your Fitness," for specifics of what kind of lifting gives what kind of results.

Have Fun

Find an active pastime you enjoy and count it as exercise. Like to go dancing? Live it up once a week and count it as one exercise class. Walk to the grocery store and carry home packages. That's two. Like to window-shop? Sightsee? Bicycle? Roller-skate? Play catch with children? Be creative.

Be Happy

Be happy. Why not?

How to Lose Fat—What to Do

- Eat low fat. Try more vegetables. Fruits make good desserts.
- See a physician skilled in nutrition and exercise.
- Find all the things that you can do in a day to be more active—without going to a gym.
- Educate yourself. Read about fitness and nutrition. Carefully choose sources with real medical information, not hype and sales pitches.

27

Cardiovascular Disease

The trouble with heart disease is that the first symptom is often hard to deal with: sudden death

—Michael Phelps, M.D.

What condition kills more people than any other? Cardiovascular disease. It's the number one noninjury cause of death beginning at age thirty for men and forty for women. Nearly half of all deaths in the United States each year are from cardiovascular disease, which includes heart attack and stroke. It kills twice as many men and women as cancer. Most men dying a sudden death during physical activity have been found to have underlying heart disease. The good news is that cardiovascular disease is largely preventable, by things you can do yourself at home.

How Does Cardiovascular Disease Affect You?

Cardiovascular disease keeps you from enjoying your life in several ways:

- It can end your life at a young age.

- It reduces your physical capacity to deal with exertion.
- It limits your ability to go out and enjoy life.
- Dealing with environmental stresses on your body from weather extremes of heat and cold are hard enough on your cardiovascular system. But cardiovascular disease greatly limits your ability to do that safely. Even men with no underlying heart disease usually display greater blood pressure and other cardiovascular responses, such as irregular heartbeats, than women during activities in the cold.
- For men who have underlying cardiovascular problems, the combination of work and cold in activities such as shoveling snow can be potentially lethal.

Cardiovascular Disease Affects More Than Just Your Heart

Your blood vessels can clog up all over your body, not just in your heart. One common place is your brain. Reduced blood flow to your brain can hurt your mental processes. "Hardening of the arteries" may explain an older person's senile behavior. An often missed warning of heart attack and stroke is confusion and change in reasoning powers.

Another interesting place is your Achilles tendon, the large "string" that attaches your calf muscle to your heel. Arteries clogged with cholesterol plaques in your Achilles tendon cause lower leg pain and problems, and predispose the area to injury, which seems to be increasingly common in middle-aged men. These injuries are more common in industrialized nations because of the link to vascular problems from Western diet and sedentary lifestyle.

Another body site also concerns men. An often ignored warning signal of dangerously narrowed arteries is decrease in erectile function. Men with this warning sign should check the possibility of cardiovascular disease with their physicians.

Risk Factors for Cardiovascular Disease

There are major and minor indicators of your chance of developing cardiovascular disease. Although some factors are more serious than others, all are cumulative, meaning the more you have, the greater your risk.

Four Top Risk Factors

Until recently there were three top risk factors:

1. Cigarette smoking.
2. High blood pressure.
3. High blood cholesterol.

Now a fourth major risk factor has been identified—no real surprise:

4. Lack of exercise.

These four are the most predictive factors of your risk.

Other Common Risk Factors

Your risk usually increases with:

- Age.
- Family history of cardiovascular problems.
- Diabetes.
- High body fat.
- How much fat you eat, particularly animal fat.
- Being male—men develop cardiovascular disease, on average, about ten years younger than women.
- Even with no other risk factors present, you may have a sudden heart attack if you use cocaine.

Too Much Iron

A recently identified and intriguing possible risk factor is high blood iron level. Iron in the body is usually found in a form tightly bound with a protein, as in hemoglobin. Iron is an oxidant and when it becomes available in unbound form, it turns on several harmful reactions with oxygen that damage your cells. People with high iron levels have been found to develop high rates of heart disease. Conversely, premenopausal women who lose small monthly amounts of iron, and vegetarians and athletes who often run a bit low, have lower incidence of heart disease than the rest of the population. High iron levels may also be linked to unusual fatigue, and possibly cancer. It's another good reason to cut back on red meat, which has a high iron content.

About 2% of all Americans have a genetic disorder that doesn't allow them to process iron, a condition called hemochromatosis. The high iron levels that they build sometimes cause heart failure. Recent news is that even slightly high iron levels may raise the risk even in those without the faulty gene, particularly men, who don't have the benefit of monthly blood loss. This seems to be more common than previously thought. James Cook, M.D., an iron specialist at the University of Kansas Medical Center states, "No one, unless he or she has been diagnosed with an iron deficiency, or belongs to a high risk group, should routinely take iron supplements." How common is this? Dr. Victor Herbert, chief of Mount Sinai's hematology and nutrition lab in the Bronx, states, "Only 6% of Americans have iron deficiency anemia. Twelve percent have a hemochromatosis related iron overload."

Not Enough Fruit and Vegetable Vitamins

Beside the well-known association between cardiovascular health and healthy eating in general, many vegetables have folic acid. Folic acid, a B vitamin, has several functions in your body. One is to lower your levels of a substance called homocysteine. Homocysteine occurs naturally in your body and has many roles. But in high amounts, it is associated with heart attack and stroke. The average meat-centered Western diet can result in deficiencies of common vitamins, including folic acid.

Folic acid deficiencies might be responsible for 15–40% of all heart attacks and strokes, depending on the study cited, a large number in either case. Eating more folic acid won't make up for a sedentary lifestyle and unhealthy eating habits, but getting enough folic acid (about 400 micrograms per day) seems to be important to cardiovascular health. Find folic acid in green leafy vegetables like spinach, Brussels sprouts, lettuce, and many fruits, including oranges and apples.

Sleep Apnea

Sleep apnea was detailed earlier in the section on the problems of overweight. "Apnea" means to stop breathing temporarily. In sleep apnea, the sleeper stops breathing, sometimes hundreds of times per night. They may make loud, labored snores and efforts to breathe. The episodes of apnea starve their bodies of oxygen. Low oxygen seems to make fatty plaques deposit in their blood vessels. Sleep apnea is a risk factor for stroke and heart attack. The many nighttime awakenings also causes chronic daytime sleepiness. This sleepiness greatly raises the risk of serious automobile accidents. Sleep apnea is a serious sleep disorder. An effective treatment for sleep apnea is losing weight.

The Four Top Risk Factors

- Cigarette smoking
- Lack of exercise
- High blood pressure
- High blood cholesterol

Other Risk Factors

- High dietary fat
- Diabetes
- High body fat
- Cocaine use
- Increasing age
- Possibly high iron
- Sleep apnea
- Being male

What Is Your Risk?

There are several pen-and-paper assessment tools to help you determine your own risk. One from the Michigan Heart Association follows on pages 288 and 289. It is one of the older assessments, but a good and easy one to start with. Circle the number in each category that best describes you. Then total your score.

Reducing Your Risk of Heart Disease

You can't do much about your age, gender, or family history. Happily, there are plenty of things you can do. Of the four major risk factors, you can directly control how much you exercise and smoke,

CARDIAC RISK INDEX

	10 to 20 **1**	21 to 30 **2**	31 to 40 **3**	41 to 50 **4**	51 to 60 **6**	61 to 70 **8**
2. Heredity	No known history **1**	One relative over 60 with cardiovascular disease **2**	Two relatives over 60 with cardiovascular disease **3**	One relative under 60 with cardiovascular disease **4**	Two relatives under 60 with cardiovascular disease **6**	Three relatives under 60 with cardiovascular disease **8**
3. Weight	More than 5 lbs below standard weight **0**	−5 to +5 lbs standard weight **1**	6–20 lbs overweight **2**	21–35 lbs overweight **3**	36–50 lbs overweight **5**	51–65 lbs overweight **7**
4. Tobacco Smoking	Nonuser **0**	Cigar and/or pipe **1**	10 cigarettes or less a day **2**	20 cigarettes a day **4**	30 cigarettes a day **6**	40 cigarettes or more a day **10**
5. Exercise	Intensive occupational and recreational exertion **1**	Moderate occupational and recreational exertion **2**	Sedentary work and intense recreational exertion **3**	Sedentary work and moderate recreational exertion **5**	Sedentary work and light recreational exertion **6**	Complete lack of all exercise **8**

	Cholesterol below 180 mg% No animal or solid fat in diet	Cholesterol 181–205 mg% 10% animal or solid fat in diet	Cholesterol 206–230 mg% 20% animal or solid fat in diet	Cholesterol 231–155 mg% 30% animal or solid fat in diet	Cholesterol 256–280 mg% 40% animal or solid fat in diet	Cholesterol 281–330 mg% 50% animal or solid fat in diet
6. Cholesterol or, if not known, % fat in the diet	1	2	3	4	5	7
7. Blood Pressure	100 upper reading **1**	120 upper reading **2**	140 upper reading **3**	160 upper reading **4**	180 upper reading **6**	200 or over upper reading **8**
8. Gender	Female under 40 **1**	Female 40–50 **2**	Female over 50 **3**	Male **5**	Stocky male **6**	Bald stocky male **7**

Total score _____

If You Score:

6–11   Your risk is well below average
12–17 Risk below average
18–24 Risk generally average
25–31 Risk moderate
32–40 Risk at a dangerous level
41–62 Danger urgent. See your physician now.

RISKO is reprinted with permission and courtesy of Michigan Heart Association © Michigan Heart Association.

and indirectly control high blood pressure, diabetes, and cholesterol with exercise, supervised medication, and healthy nutrition. Most cardiovascular disease has a large nutrition and fitness component. You can reduce your risk through healthy eating and exercise habits.

Adopt Healthy Habits

You've heard it before. Exercise more, quit smoking, and eat less sugar and fat. It gets easier the more you do it. Many fatty foods are an acquired taste. After switching to low-fat foods for a while, you'll be surprised to find how greasy the fatty foods taste when you try them again. When you eat fewer sweets, you crave them less. You'll also notice your weight and blood pressure drop if they were previously high, further reducing your risk. If you have diabetes, you can usually reduce its severity with better nutrition and more exercise. You win all around.

Start Healthy Habits Young

It's not just older people that get heart disease. Autopsies on American soldiers killed in Vietnam and Korea showed that the majority already had moderately advanced atherosclerosis. Autopsies of children who die of causes other than cardiovascular disease reveal that artery clogging can begin as early as childhood, the product of a sedentary lifestyle and the modern diet of chips, fries, burgers, and ice cream. Habits developed early, both good and bad, are more likely to be kept throughout your life.

Clogged arteries begin in youth. Heart disease is not just something that happens suddenly to older people.

Eat More Fruits and Vegetables

Make vegetables more of the main part of your meals, and less of being just side dishes. Fruit can make easy and good-tasting snacks and desserts. See your physician, registered dietitian, or exercise physiologist for a program to cut dietary fat and learn how to eat more healthfully.

Lower Your Blood Cholesterol

Two thirds of all heart attacks happen to people with cholesterol readings over 200. The average cholesterol reading in the United States is around 220. Cholesterol poses a double hazard. It slowly deposits on blood vessel walls, and makes blood vessels more likely to suddenly squeeze shut, contributing to ministrokes that warn of serious illness to come. Your blood cholesterol can rise with eating high amounts of cholesterol, and by eating lots of saturated fats.

Cholesterol is found only in animal products such as eggs, dairy, and meat. Your liver makes all the cholesterol you need. You don't have to eat any at all. For more on cholesterol, see the next chapter. The amount of saturated fat you eat relates to your blood cholesterol levels. Cutting back on saturated fat helps reduce your risk of high cholesterol. Saturated fats are mostly found in meat, dairy, and hydrogenated vegetable oils.

Consider Estrogen After Menopause

After surgical or natural menopause, a woman's risk of cardiovascular disease soars until just about matching that of a man. Estrogen replacement reduces a woman's chance of heart attack by about half. Speak with your physician about the benefits and risks of estrogen replacement that apply to your current state of health.

Pick Up the Phone

An easy thing to do. Call your physician to ask how to reduce your risk. If you don't have a personal physician, call a physician referral service to find a physician that fits your needs and likes.

Donate Blood

Some experts recommend regular blood donations to avoid high blood iron levels that may relate to disease risk. This usually is only for certain people with abnormally high iron levels. The *British Medical Journal* reports on a study from Finland of 2,600 men. Nearly 10% of the men who had not donated blood in the two previous years suffered a heart attack. Only 1 of the 153 who had donated blood had a heart attack in the same period of time. Although it is possible that the men who had donated blood were more health conscious in general, the connection in the study seemed to be strong. Call your local Red Cross for information on donating blood—to help someone who needs blood, and possibly yourself.

Get in Better Physical Shape

Being out of shape is a vicious cycle. You are not able to do enough exercise to improve your health. So you become more out of shape, and unhealthier. Your risk of a problem brought on by exertion rises. Being in better shape lowers your risk of cardiovascular disease while exercising, and improves your ability to do the amount of exercise you need to become healthier.

Have a Social Support Network

Behavioral researchers report that having a social structure of friends is heart-healthy. Speculated reasons include that friends share health information, and that the support of friendship reduces physical and emotional stress. Many people socially isolate themselves. How can they develop a better network of friends? Writer and philosopher Ralph Waldo Emerson observed, "If you would have a friend, you must first be one." Make time for friends, accept people as they are, and respect their secrets. That will go a long way to developing and keeping friendships.

Know the Symptoms of a Heart Attack

If you get chest pain, chest tightness, shortness of breath, or pain down one arm, go immediately to a hospital emergency department. Don't dismiss these warnings as indigestion. Don't ignore these symptoms in a woman. Cardiovascular disease is the number one disease of both women and men.

Get Medical Care Right Away

Even if the pain goes away, it doesn't necessarily mean you didn't have a heart attack. How well the hospital can care for you if you are having a heart attack depends on how quickly you get there. Delay reduces the effectiveness of the many treatment options available. Quick treatment (within six hours) prevents more extensive, irreversible damage to your heart. Call for help instead of trying to get to an emergency room yourself. Some people have a full-out attack while driving to the hospital, and never make it there. Call ahead to your doctor to meet you there.

Reduce Your Risk of Heart Disease

- Adopt healthy habits. Exercise more, quit smoking, and eat less sugar and fat.
- Start healthy habits young. Habits developed early, both good and bad, are more likely to be kept throughout your life.
- Eat more fruits and vegetables.
- Lower your blood cholesterol by exercising more, and eating less saturated fat.
- Consider estrogen replacement. Heart attack risk rises sharply after menopause. Estrogen replacement reduces a woman's chance of heart attack by about half.
- Call your physician or physician referral service to find a physician. Find out how to reduce your risk through healthy exercise, health, and nutrition plans.
- Donate blood. It's not certain, but possible that regular blood donations to avoid high blood iron levels that may increase disease risk.
- Get in better physical shape. Being in better shape lowers your risk of cardiovascular disease while exercising, and improves your ability to do the amount of exercise you need to become healthier.
- Know the symptoms of heart attack.
- Have a support network of real friends.
- Get medical care right away. If you get chest pain, chest tightness, shortness of breath, or pain down one arm, go immediately to a hospital emergency department.

Be Proactive, Not Reactive

The reactive approach is to sit around, get clogged blood vessels, wait for the physician to prescribe drugs, worry, have surgery, have a stroke, have a heart attack. Your heredity is not your destiny. If your father had heart disease, you're not doomed. On the other hand, the more common approach is "My father (or mother) didn't have heart disease, so I have nothing to worry about." Neither is completely true. Be proactive with preventive care. Cardiovascular disease develops largely through unhealthy habits making it, fortunately, largely preventable.

Resources for More Information

AMERICAN HEART ASSOCIATION
National Center
7272 Greenville Ave.
Dallas, TX 75231-4596
(800) 242-8721
(214) 373-6300

AMERICAN RED CROSS
For referral to a CPR class near you, call (800) 42-CROSS.

IRON OVERLOAD DISEASES ASSOCIATION
433 Westwind Drive
Palm Beach, FL 33408
(888) 678-4766

28

Good and Bad Cholesterol Explained

Avoid fried meats, which angry up the blood.

—Rule 1 of the 6 Rules of Staying Young
by Satchel Paige

You're going out for the day. Got your keys? Check. Jacket? Check. Wallet? Check. Favorable lipoprotein ratio?

What Is a Lipoprotein?

You've probably heard of the different kinds of lipoproteins as "good cholesterol" and "bad cholesterol." Lipoproteins aren't just cholesterol. Lipoproteins are large molecules that your body makes out of cholesterol, fat (lipid), and protein. Lipids won't dissolve in your blood or travel through your blood on their own, so they have to be carried around by helpful proteins.

There are five kinds of lipoproteins. This chapter covers two: high-density lipoprotein, or HDL (good cholesterol), and low-density lipoprotein, or LDL (bad cholesterol).

Lipoproteins and Cholesterol

Cholesterol is one of three lipids ushered around your blood by lipoproteins. Cholesterol is a necessary ingredient in your body. Why? It is a precursor of your steroid hormones, including all your sex hormones, and a precursor of your bile acids, which handle fat digestion. Your body uses it to make Vitamin D, and it is a necessary part of every cell membrane in your body.

In excess, cholesterol deserves its bad reputation. Too much cholesterol in cells lining your arteries builds up deposits called atherosclerotic plaques (*athero* means "gruel-like," and *sclerosis* means "hardening"). About a third of all American adults have cholesterol readings high enough to indicate a high risk of heart disease. According to physician Dr. Dean Ornish, the "average" American has a cholesterol reading around 220, and the average American develops heart disease. Dr. Ornish is known for his work with reducing heart disease with a program that includes very low dietary fat.

"Bad" Lipoproteins and Heart Disease

Low-density lipoprotein is called "bad cholesterol" for a good reason. Fatty plaques that narrow blood vessels are made of LDL and VLDL (very low-density lipoproteins).

LDL picks up 60–75% of the cholesterol from the fats you eat and from your liver, which makes cholesterol, and takes it to the cells of your blood vessels and muscles. Because LDL carries most of the cholesterol, a high amount of LDL in your blood translates to a higher risk of heart attack and angina pectoris (*angina* means "pain," and *pectoris* "chest").

What "Good" Lipoproteins Do

High-density lipoprotein (HDL), popularly called good cholesterol, removes cholesterol from your bloodstream, and does not collect or stick to the inner linings of your arteries. HDL contains an enzyme that helps break down deposits, and takes "used" cholesterol away from the cells back to your liver for recycling and excretion. The higher your HDL level, the lower your risk of heart disease.

Figure 28.1. You don't eat bad cholesterol, or low-density lipoproteins (LDLs); your body makes them. Your body can wind up with too much LDL when you eat too much animal fat or saturated vegetable fat, smoke, take drugs such as anabolic steroids, and don't exercise.

Dr. David Hsu, of the University of Iowa Hospitals and Clinics, describes the 4 main functions of HDL:

- "It is an airport baggage handler that tags and de-tags chylomicrons, VLDL's and IDL's (the very low and intermediate density guys) with protein tags that identifies them and allows them to be picked up out of your blood (the conveyor belt) by the correct recipient at the correct destination. The tags are called apoproteins.
- It is a maintenance person, picking up garbage (free cholesterol) from peripheral tissue (e.g., from cell membranes of dead or live cells) and stores them, using an enzyme that makes the cholesterol even more willing to stay inside the HDL maintenance person.
- It is a porter that carries cholesterol back to the liver, where the HDL is broken down and the cholesterol released into liver cells to be used as needed.
- It is a trader, and trades cholesterol stores with VLDL's and LDL's for fats.

Vegetable Oil • High Density Lipoproteins • Health • Slim

HDLs

Figure 28.2. You can increase your good cholesterol, or high-density lipoprotein (HDL) level, by avoiding smoking, avoiding drugs such as anabolic steroids, eating less animal fat and more vegetables, and exercising more.

What Distinguishes High from Low Density?

The names "high" and "low density" come from two characteristics of lipoproteins. The first is lipid content. LDL has more lipid than HDL. Normally when you call something "low," you think of a smaller amount. But the higher lipid content of LDL decreases the density because fat is less dense than other body constituents. Think of cream floating on milk. Heavy cream has more fat than light cream, making it less dense. Although it weighs less than light cream, it's called heavy for its higher fat content. In the same way LDL has more fat but lower density.

The names "high" and "low" also come from the way they're packaged. Loosely packed LDL cholesterol floats through the bloodstream to your cells. Cholesterol released from the cells tightly crams into HDL for the voyage back to your liver.

Physical therapist Marla Tonseth offers this way to remember which is which:

HDL = **H**ealthy
LDL = **L**ousy

How to Get Less LDL and More HDL

Improving your ratio of good to bad cholesterol is not so difficult. Lipoproteins ferry LDL and HDL to and from each cell in amounts determined by your food choices and activity level. Although blood vessel diseases like heart attack and stroke are the number one killers in the United States and Great Britain, they are practically strangers in half the world. In those areas, intake of animal products and fat is low, activity level is high, and smoking is almost unknown.

Less Saturated Fat and Cholesterol

LDL levels may be directly related to eating saturated fat, although the question of how much dietary fat intake affects the pattern of HDL and LDL cholesterol levels has not been answered for certain. It is agreed that saturated fat increases the rate of cholesterol formation, and that people, especially those at risk of heart disease, who already have a heart condition, or are overweight, should limit cholesterol, and more importantly, saturated fat in their food.

You get saturated fat from all animal sources like meat, fowl, dairy, and eggs. In contrast, vegetable oils are not saturated except tropical palm and coconut oils. Beware of ingredients in packaged foods like hydrogenated vegetable oils. Hydrogenation artificially saturates vegetable oil.

Cholesterol is part of every cell membrane in animals, giving the outer cell area part of the structure it needs. Plants don't need cholesterol around their cells, because they have rigid cell walls. That's why only animal products have cholesterol. There's no need for you to eat cholesterol to get the amount your body needs to do its job. Your liver manufactures all you need—even if you eat no cholesterol at all.

Quit Smoking

If there weren't already enough reasons for you to quit smoking, here's another: Smoking lowers HDL.

Avoid Anabolic Steroids

The male hormone testosterone depresses HDL levels, one reason men's risk of heart disease is higher than women's risk. Taking extra male hormones called anabolic steroids plummets HDL levels.

Exercise

Exercise more effectively changes HDL/LDL ratio than dietary change and weight loss. Endurance exercise increases HDL and its important enzyme, and decreases total blood cholesterol and LDL in both men and women. An altered blood lipid profile may be one of the principal mechanisms of a reduced risk of heart disease through exercise.

Several studies published in well-accepted medical journals report that more exercise and less dietary cholesterol and fat may not only stop coronary artery disease from progressing, but reverse it.

How to Lower Your "Bad Cholesterol"

- Eat less saturated fat and cholesterol.
- Quit smoking.
- Avoid anabolic steroids.
- Exercise more.

Your Cholesterol Ratio

Your total cholesterol reading is determined by your LDL and HDL levels. You raise your risk of heart disease if you have too much total cholesterol, and if you have too little good cholesterol (HDL). High levels of circulating HDL in relation to LDL are usually more important than your total amount of blood cholesterol.

Your total, and the ratio of good to total, is a number easily determined by blood testing. In general, the lower your cholesterol ratio, the lower your risk of heart disease.

Before an Exercise and Low-Fat Diet Program:

$$\frac{\text{total cholesterol } 200}{\text{good (HDL) cholesterol } 50} = 4.0$$

This is a high ratio. The optimal ratio is 3.5 or lower.

After a Program to Raise Good Cholesterol:

$$\frac{\text{total cholesterol } 180}{\text{good (HDL) cholesterol } 60} = 3.0$$

This is a good ratio. Optimal ratio is 3.5 or lower.

Occasionally, people who eat very low-fat diets, particularly vegetarian diets, lower their LDL level so much that their cholesterol ratio becomes high. This should not be mistaken for an unfavorable ratio. These people have a lower-than-average risk of heart disease. The big picture of blood fats is what is important.

A Priority

Much attention is paid to the few yearly deaths by sensational events such as plane crashes. At the same time, hundreds of thousands of people die every year by the frying pan. Heart disease is still the Number One killer of both men and women. What will change that, more than any drug or fad health food, are healthy food choices and regular exercise. So get rid of the cigarettes, get more vegetables on your plate, and get exercising.

Resources for More Information

AMERICAN HEART ASSOCIATION
National Center
7272 Greenville Ave.
Dallas, TX 75231-4596
(800) 242-8721
(214) 373-6300

29

Headaches

One man's food is another man's poison.

—Socrates

Foods or actions that cause no pain to some people can trigger a terrible headache in others. Two thousand years ago, physicians required their patients to fast as part of their medical exams. Often, the patients' symptoms would stop.

Many headaches are caused by things you can change, meaning that many headaches are preventable. This section is not intended for use as a medical diagnosis, and is by no means complete, but is a look at possible mechanisms and things to do for relief.

Types of Headaches

There seems to be a continuum between the various kinds of headaches, particularly tension-type and migraine. These types of headaches may represent ends of a single continuum rather than being distinct from one another. Modern headache centers take an integrated approach to understanding the types of headaches, leading to better diagnosis and treatment. The types of headaches are described here separately to introduce them in an organized fashion.

Tension-Type Headaches

Previously called muscle contraction headaches, or tension headaches, these can occur when you tense the muscles of your face, brow, scalp, and neck for lengthy periods. For example, frowning and brow furrowing over taxes or other stressful paperwork; tensing over a desk, computer, or workbench; shouldering the phone to your ear, clenching your teeth. The pain is steady, felt on one or both sides of the head, or can often feel like a tight band around the head. Since tension headaches are often triggered by stressing the head and neck muscles for long periods of time, tension headaches typically start late in the day, and resolve with sleep. Tension headaches usually disappear after the stress is over, but if you habitually tense your muscles day after day, you can have pain from it day after day.

Migraines

The pain of migraine headaches is thought to result from inflammation of the blood vessels surrounding the brain. Nausea, vomiting, and sensitivity to light and sound may occur. The pain can be so terrible that even a word meaning "depression or unhappiness" (*megrems*) comes from a Middle English variant of migraine.

Migraine can occur with or without an "aura"—neurological symptoms appearing 10 to 30 minutes before a classic migraine. An aura may include flashing or zigzag lights, lines, and dots, dimmed vision, tingling in the face or hands, weakness of an arm or leg, speech difficulties, or confusion. Migraine usually starts on one side of the head and may spread to the other side. Left untreated, attacks can last up to three intensely painful days.

Migraine without aura used to be called common migraine, because it is more common than migraine with aura. When warnings occur, they might include fatigue, mental fuzziness, mood changes, or unusual fluid retention. These symptoms, as well as those of the aura, indicate that the generator of migraine is in the brain, not the blood vessels. Untreated, common migraine pain can last up to three days. If it lasts longer, it is called migraine status.

There are several other kinds of migraine. Hemiplegic migraine produces temporary paralysis on one side of the body (hemiplegia). Basilar artery migraine (named for a problem in a major brain artery called the basilar artery) is often seen in young women. In ophthalmoplegic migraine, the pain is around the eye and causes droopy eyelids and double vision.

Dr. William B. Young, of the Jefferson Headache Center in Philadelphia, explains migraine origins. "Ten to fifteen years ago, it was state of the art to say that migraine began with changes in brain blood vessels. Today, we have evidence that migraine sufferers have a lowered threshold of the "migraine generator" within the brain. One theory is that this generator is in the brainstem, involving serotonin cells. Another theory is that an aura, or an aura-like phenomenon in the cortex of the brain, starts a cascade of events that leads to migraine pain including inflammation of the blood vessels surrounding the brain."

Cluster Headaches

These headaches are rare, but so painful, and have such a characteristic pattern, that they deserve mention. They occur mostly in men. Cluster headache sufferers experience severe bouts of pain on one side of the head for about an hour, one to three times per day. Often, cluster headaches occur at the same time every day, "clustered" into a period of weeks or months, then disappear for months to years, only to recur. Eye tearing, lid drooping, and nasal stuffiness are characteristic. Sufferers may pace, bang their heads, rock, and become irritable during the attack. The pain can be so intense, it has been called the "suicide headache."

Neurologist Jim Burke, M.D., at Albert Einstein Medical Center in Philadelphia, explains cluster headaches, "These headaches are different than migraine headaches. People who are experiencing a cluster headache will be pacing the floor holding their head, while a person experiencing a migraine will look for a dark, quiet room."

Traction and Inflammatory Headaches

These come from a variety of other problems, from stroke to sinus infection. Traction headaches can result from pulling, stretching, or pushing pain-sensitive parts of the head, for example, with tight hats, collars, and hair barrettes. Inflammatory headaches may come from elsewhere in the body, signaling problems like meningitis, trigeminal neuralgia, glaucoma, tooth infections, or problems of the sinuses.

Common Headache Triggers

Many things common in your everyday life can trigger headaches. Responses to triggers are individual. Here are a few.

Head and Neck Posture

A very common, and very overlooked, cause of tension headache is poor back and neck posture. Holding your head forward of the midline of your body is called a "forward head." The weight of your head, held in front of your neck rather than over it fatigues and strains neck muscles, overstretches the ligament down the back of your neck, and puts pressure on your cervical discs. Pain from a forward head is usually felt down the back of the head and neck, along the top of the shoulders, between the shoulders, under the lower point of the shoulder blade.

Many people have a forward head without knowing it. A forward head is accentuated if you crane your neck while driving, using computers, or watching TV. Many exercises common in gyms make a forward head worse: pulling your neck forward for abdominal work, craning and tensing your neck while lifting weights, and tipping your neck forward while lifting or pulling a bar in back of your neck. (Healthier substitutes for these exercises are in Chapter 9, "Good and Bad Exercises." A forward head is easily prevented with proper posture. Bring your head into healthy alignment by holding your ears above your shoulders, rather than letting your head crane forward of the midline of your body. More on how to correct a forward head is in Chapters 20 and 21 on back and neck pain.)

Food

For migraines, it is unusual for food to be the only trigger, but food is often part of the cause. Classic food triggers are chocolate, red wine, beer, walnuts, peanuts, liver pâté, yogurt, lima beans, and aged cheeses like bleu cheese. These foods contain the chemical tyramine, which constricts arteries, the first step to getting a migraine. The difficulty in finding out which foods are problems is that migraines often take a day or two to "bloom" after eating trigger foods. By then the connection is long forgotten.

Other headaches come from processed meats, like hot dogs. Processed meats contain nitrite compounds, which can dilate blood vessels in susceptible people, causing pounding head pain. Other times, specific foods can set off an allergic reaction, resulting in headache. If avoiding certain foods does not reduce the number of headaches you get, resume your regular diet. Don't become a "migraine hermit."

Alcohol

Nonmigraine headache is common after too much wine, whisky, brandy, or rum, because these drinks (unlike vodkas) are high in headache-causing substances called congeners. Migraine and cluster headaches are different from alcohol hangovers but may occur with a hangover, because they can both result from drinking alcohol. Cluster headaches may start shortly after a drink is taken.

Caffeine

Sometimes too much caffeine can cause a headache. But for people who habitually drink caffeine drinks, caffeine withdrawal can bring on a headache, which is a vicious cycle among some coffee and soda drinkers. Some coffee drinkers find that they will have a headache until their morning coffee, making it difficult to cut back or quit drinking coffee.

Sleep

A classic nonfood trigger for migraine is altered sleep schedules, such as sleeping later than usual. Napping with your head propped on the arm of the couch can trigger some back-of-the-head headaches.

Sleep apnea, a sleep disorder where the sleeper stops breathing, sometimes hundreds of times per night, drops oxygen levels. Many physical problems result. People suffering sleep apnea have daytime sleepiness, and often wake up headachy from the many periods of oxygen starvation. Loud snoring and gasping are clues to sleep apnea, which occurs most often among very overweight people. *See* Chapter 27, "Cardiovascular Disease," for more on sleep apnea.

Eyestrain

Close work, an eyeglass prescription that is not just right, and glare are often factors in starting a headache from eyestrain. To reduce chance of eyestrain, remember to look up and at a distance away from your work regularly, to let your eyes focus on different distances. If you wear glasses, have your glasses prescription checked. Make sure it is the right strength for you, and that all the other considerations of grinding the glass for your prescription have been faithfully met. Make sure that the distance between the pupils of your eyes was measured correctly, then ground correctly into your lenses. Ask your optometrist or optician to check the base curve and axis of your lenses. Make sure your glasses fit properly, and are the right distance from your eyes. If you don't wear glasses, have a good eye exam to see if you need correction, and to check the health of your visual system.

Less Common But Still Important Contributors

Tight Hats

Cold weather can make your head hurt. Wearing a tight hat can also cause a headache, producing a type of tension headache sometimes known as "hatus-too-tightis."

Carbon Monoxide Poisoning

Headache is a common flag of an uncommon problem—carbon monoxide poisoning. This can come from a faulty heating system at home, exhaust system in your car, blocked chimneys, or using kerosene heaters indoors. People have been poisoned by riding in the back of trailered boats or recreational vehicles. You can't smell, taste, or see carbon monoxide. Carbon monoxide poisoning can be serious, even fatal. Small, inexpensive home carbon monoxide detectors are available in stores, usually next to the smoke detectors. Make sure your home has good ventilation.

Drugs

Regular, long-term use of pain-suppressing drugs, both prescription and nonprescription, lowers your own body's natural pain-suppressing ability. Sudden withdrawal from these drugs can rebound you into a headache.

Hyperventilation

Sometimes, people begin to breathe too deeply and quickly for any number of reasons including fear and excitement. Such breathing quickly lowers body carbon dioxide levels, sometimes enough to cause limb tingling, dizziness, lightheadedness, headache, or other odd sensations.

Teeth and Jaw

Toothaches start some headaches. Biting, grinding, and clenching teeth at night during sleep can cause jaw fatigue and sometimes head pain. Poorly fitting dentures can cause jaw misalignment and pain. Someone with a dysfunction of the jaw joint, called the temporomandibular joint (TMJ), may become headachy from chronic clenching at night, or even chewing food day after day.

Sinusitis

When one or more of your sinus cavities fill with bacterial or viral fluid and become inflamed, you have sinusitis. The infection may start in your upper respiratory tract and spread to your sinuses. Sinusitis may involve allergies to irritants such as cigarette smoke, dust, ragweed, and animal hair. According to the NIH, "Research scientists disagree about whether chronic sinusitis triggers headache."

Nitroglycerin

People who get angina pectoris (meaning "chest pain" in Latin) are often prescribed nitroglycerin pills or patches to wear. Nitroglycerin dilates blood vessels, which improves blood flow and oxygenation, relieving chest pain. The nitroglycerin is important to relieving chest pain, but users often get headaches because brain blood vessels dilate, too.

A Dynamite Headache Story

Nitroglycerin is an explosive used to make dynamite and blasting gelatin. It is also used in medicine to reduce chest pain. Now who made such a connection, and what does that have to do with headaches?

The story goes that World War II dynamite factory workers endured throbbing headaches as an occupational hazard. When they left their positions after the war, their headaches stopped but some of them began dying of heart attacks. Why was this?

People whose blood vessels are narrowed by fatty deposits can't get enough blood to their heart, reducing their oxygen supply. Their heart must pump harder against narrowed areas, increasing oxygen demand. When oxygen supply doesn't meet oxygen demand, their heart cries out in pain, called angina pectoris. A physician may prescribe nitroglycerin, which dilates the blood vessels of the heart, restoring blood flow and relieving pain. It also dilates the blood vessels of the head. Headaches are a characteristic symptom of too much nitro.

Nitrates are the active ingredient in nitroglycerin. Munitions workers had been inhaling airborne nitrates on the job, sometimes causing headaches but also dilating their coronary blood vessels. After discontinuing exposure, the vasodilatory effect was rapidly lost. Their blood vessels constricted to their previous size. Headaches vanished. But those workers with coronary vessels already diseased from the usual causes—high-fat diet and lack of exercise, fell victim to blocked blood flow to their hearts. By leaving the ordnance plants they lost the protective vasodilatory effect of their workplace air.

Nitroglycerin is very explosive. Dynamite is close to 75% nitroglycerin. Because it is mixed with inert materials like sawdust, wood pulp, or diatomaceous earth, it will detonate only with a fuse or the kick of a blasting cap. But medicinal nitroglycerin will not blow up because is only about 1% nitroglycerin and is packed in an absorbent, inert material that reduces its volatility. Just watch out for headaches.

Other Contributors

Headaches can come from allergies, air pollution, bright sunshine, hunger, thirst, cigarette smoke, dust, and fumes from chemicals and paint. "Benign exertional headaches" can occur when starting physical activity, such as running, lifting, and even coughing, sneezing, or bending. These headaches are more common in men, and rarely last more than a few minutes. Fatigue, glaring, or flickering lights, even changes in the weather can set off headaches.

Combinations of Things

Determining what triggers your headaches can be tricky. Often it is a combination of things that singly would do little to cause pain. For example, you may endure a tough day, a high smog count, an uncomfortable office chair or car seat, and too much coffee because you didn't sleep well the previous night. Then you go out for dinner that night and have red wine and a chocolate dessert. That might be the final straw producing a killer migraine the next day.

Treating Headaches

During the Stone Age, medical shamans treated headaches by cutting holes in the patient's skull with flints to let the demons out. The term for this practice is trephination. Not only did patients survive trephination, it seemed to be popular. Some skulls unearthed from that period show more than one healed trephine hole. By the ninth century, a headache remedy from the British Isles was to drink "the juice of elderseed, cow's brain, and goat's dung dissolved in vinegar."

Understandably, headache sufferers often will do almost anything to relieve the terrible pain. Fortunately, today there are better remedies.

Tension-Type Headaches

Ordinary muscle-triggered headaches go away when you stop tensing your face, head, and neck. Acute muscle-contraction headaches can be relieved with a hot shower or moist heat, and over-the-counter pain relievers like Tylenol®. Training for better head and neck posture can reduce much of the pain that is common down the back of the neck, into the shoulder blades, and along the tops of the shoulders (*see* Chapters 20 and 21 on back and neck pain). Physical therapy and gentle exercise of the neck may be helpful. Pushing your fingers against the forehead, from brows to hairline, slowly, repeatedly, and firmly, seems to be a helpful massage for tension headache.

Some people have fierce tensing habits, triggering chronic headaches. They need to retrain their postural habits, and learn not to tense their muscles. They can do this through good physical therapy and exercises, and the various kinds of biofeedback, relaxation training, and counseling.

Migraine Headaches

According to neurologist and headache specialist Dr. William Young, the most commonly prescribed drugs used to relieve migraines are ergotamine tartrate, DHE, and sumatriptan. They can be taken at the beginning of a migraine to stop it cold. Combination medicines containing Excedrin®, Midrin®, or Fiurnal® can be effective. Dr. Young stresses the importance of not overusing pain medications (more than 2–3 days a week) or a daily rebound headache may result. Rebound headaches can be severe enough to require hospitalization.

During a migraine, it helps to seek a dark, quiet room, and use cold packs. Sometimes it helps to press on the bulging artery in front of the ear on the painful side.

Cluster Headaches

Medications commonly prescribed for cluster headache include drugs like caferget, DHE, and sumatriptan. Since one of the mechanisms proposed for at least one stage of cluster headache is enlarged and inflamed brain blood vessels, various treatments aim to reduce the size of the enlarged blood vessels using ice hats or oxygen. When you breathe pure oxygen, your body constricts brain blood vessels to protect your brain from the ill effects of too high levels of oxygen. Breathing 100% oxygen has been known to help relieve some cases of headache, but there are very little good data on this. Breathing oxygen at higher than usual pressures in a hyperbaric chamber is also under study. Most people with cluster headaches require medication. Pain medications rarely work, but more specific treatments are successful in the vast majority.

Trigeminal Neuralgia

Also called tic douloureux (painful tic), this condition can cause brief, "lightning bolts" of facial pain, set off by the smallest touch or movement of the face or mouth. It comes from a problem of a facial nerve called the trigeminal nerve. This nerve supplies your face, teeth, mouth, and nose with sensation, and also lets you chew. People with trigeminal neuralgia may fear chewing or brushing their teeth because those actions can set off the pain.

Treatment for trigeminal neuralgia involves various medications, taken regularly for prevention. In other cases, surgery directly on the trigeminal nerve can stop the episodes.

Acute and Chronic Sinusitis

Home treatments include hot facial compresses, sniffing salt water mixtures to reduce irritation and swelling, pain relievers, decongestants, and keeping your home free of allergens (shag rugs, cats, whatever the trigger irritant). In addition to over-the-counter decongestants, some people get rapid results with spicy foods and hot peppers. Others take steam baths. Medical treatment may involve allergy shots, vasoconstrictors, and inhaled steroids to shrink swollen inflamed membranes allowing better drainage, other compounds that reduce the amount of inflammation-causing histamine released, and occasionally, antibiotics if the problem is bacterial.

When to See a Physician

Many headaches don't require medical care. Headaches from the occasional missed meal, muscle tension, or poor posture are easily remedied. But some headaches signal serious problems such as head injury, stroke, or disease. According to the National Institutes of Health, you need prompt medical care for the following:

- Sudden, severe headache (reaching a maximum in less than one minute).
- Headache associated with convulsions.
- Headache accompanied by confusion or loss of consciousness.
- Headache following a blow to the head.
- Headache associated with pain in the eye or ear.

- Persistent headache in a person who was previously headache-free.
- Recurring headache in children.
- Headache associated with fever.
- Headache that interferes with normal life.

Preventing Headaches

To avoid tension-type headaches, good posture is important. Check to see if you hold your head in a forward posture (*see* Chapters 20 and 21, "Back and Neck Pain"). Avoid teeth clenching and grinding. Look in the mirror to see if you habitually purse your lips, furrow your brow, squint, or look surprised. Relax and enjoy your day. Some people keep a mirror at their desk to catch candid reflections when they are not "posing" for a mirror.

Figure 29.1. A tension-type headache in the making.

Common methods to prevent migraine headaches include medications, biofeedback training, stress reduction, regular exercise, and eliminating trigger foods and activities. To find food triggers, keep a food diary. For one week, write down every food you eat, and the time of day. In the same space, note how you feel. Also log the weather, what work and exercise you did that day, and anything else you think may relate. Review your food/headache journal after one week (or longer if you did not have a headache during that time). Look for what happened in the 24 to 48 hours before your headache.

Some migraine patients need preventive medications, taken daily,which can begin to control headaches in three to six weeks. Vitamin B₂ (riboflavin) has been shown effective for some migraine sufferers. The dose is 400 milligrams a day, a very high dose, although with few reported side effects. Your physician can determine which migraine treatment, or combination of treatments, is right for you.

Finding the cause is important to ending inflammatory and other headaches. For example, headaches from temporomandibular joint (TMJ) problems can be corrected with devices for the mouth, and retraining chewing habits.

See your physician for assessment to identify what kinds of headache you get and what usually triggers it. Take a good look at your posture, nutrition, exercise, physical condition, and surroundings. Have your teeth and eyes checked. Have your furnace and chimneys checked. Find out if you tense your face and neck. Find out if you have allergies. Keep a list of what you eat to see if you have any trigger foods. Then, as obvious as it sounds, work to avoid things that give you headaches.

Resources for More Information

NATIONAL HEADACHE FOUNDATION
Toll-free hot line (800) 843-2256

AMERICAN COUNCIL FOR HEADACHE EDUCATION (ACHE) NEWSLETTER
Suite 200
875 Kings Highway
West Deptford, NJ 08096

30

Leg Cramps and What to Do About Them

For this, be sure, to-night thou shalt have cramps,
Side-stitches that shall pen thy breath up; urchins
Shall, for that vast of night that they may work,
All exercise on thee; thou shalt be pinch'd
As thick as honeycomb, each pinch more stinging
Than bees that made 'em.

—Prospero, in *The Tempest,* Act I, Scene II

What Are Leg Cramps?

Muscles contract to move your bones. That's their job. The muscles that move your bones around are voluntary muscles. You tell them when to contract. After you stop telling them, they relax. When a muscle contracts too much, too suddenly, and does not relax again, that is a cramp. It is a spasm. It hurts. Leg cramps usually occur in your calf, foot, or hamstring muscles, but occasionally affect the quadriceps muscles in the front of your thigh, or other muscles.

Calf Cramps

Your gastrocnemius, or calf muscle, is the prominent, fleshy muscle at the back of your lower leg, below your knee. It attaches from your knee to your heel. Its main job is to pull on your heel to point your foot down, an action called plantarflexion. Plantarflexion flexes your ankle toward the sole, or plantar surface of your foot. You can (usually) easily see the "string" that your calf muscle attaches to your heel to pull with. The string is a tendon called the Achilles tendon. When your calf muscle cramps, it pulls your Achilles tendon abnormally strongly and won't let go, which pulls your foot downward into a pointed (plantar flexed) position, and holds it there painfully.

Foot Cramps

Your foot muscles that curl your toes down extend along the bottom of your foot from your heel to your toes. When these muscles cramp, they pull your toes, usually your two middle ones, downward toward the sole of your foot—painfully—and hold them there in spasm.

Upper Leg Cramps

A hamstring cramp will hurt in the back of your upper leg, and contract your hamstring muscles enough to make your knee bend. A quadriceps cramp will tighten the front of your thigh, causing your leg to straighten out, painfully.

Why?

There is one very common reason why people get cramps in their calves and feet, and several uncommon reasons for cramps in general. First the less common reasons:

People like to say that not eating enough salt, or bananas, or any particular food causes leg cramps, but that is an unlikely reason. In Western societies, a deficiency of salt or potassium is hard to get. The average Westerner eats many times the amount needed, and the body helpfully "pees" it all out until levels are normalized again. Biochemical reasons why an overstressed muscle may cramp are not pinned down. Scientists would love to know the chemistry, too. Some people may get cramps from too much salt or potassium loss because of disease, diuretics, or large fluid losses from prolonged vomiting or diarrhea. But it seems that in the general population, muscle cramps during exercise are not from large electrolyte disturbances.

An uncommon cause of constant, severe calf cramps is cirrhosis of the liver. A rare possibility is certain inherited disorders that specifically cause leg cramps. Sometimes the pain is not muscle cramps at all, but from other conditions confused for cramps. Arteries of the leg can plug up for the same reasons blood vessels anywhere in the body plug up—vascular disease is not just of the heart. When a person with narrowed leg arteries starts activity, the legs need more blood than can fit through those vessels, and the leg cries in pain for oxygen. That is called claudication, from a Latin word meaning "lameness." Those at highest risk are sedentary, smokers, or fond of high-fat diets. Another issue is pregnancy, which often presses on vessels exiting to the legs, causing leg pain and cramping.

Those are some uncommon reasons for leg cramps. Now what is the usual reason?

The Most Common Reason

Foot and leg cramps are often caused by holding your leg, ankle, and foot muscles tightly, rather than letting them swing fluidly when you walk around all day. Tight shoes that restrict your toes or the natural range of motion of your foot when walking change the way your legs need to move, and can shorten the muscles into being more cramp-ready. The extra work of tensing the muscle makes it overexert, another factor in cramping.

You can get leg cramps from holding your leg, ankle, and foot muscles tightly, rather than letting them swing fluidly during walking.

Calf cramps during swimming are most usually caused by kicking with tight ankles, and holding the foot at a rigid angle. The rigid, unyielding way the foot and leg are held overstresses the muscles trying to do the work of moving you. Cramps at the bottom of the foot are usually from kicking with toes curled or hooked. Tightly hooked toes, either by habit, or finning in fins too large or too small, tightly contracts the muscles at the bottom of the foot, which easily go into spasm. Sometimes a swimmer will bend the knees too much, too hard while finning, overstressing the hamstrings, the muscles at the back of the thigh, causing them to cramp as well. In a pool, pushing too hard off the wall to do a start or turn can contract the calf muscle too tightly, making it cramp.

The most common reason swimmers get leg cramps is
kicking with tight ankles and hooked toes.

What to Do

Relieving a cramp can be easy and quick. A cramp is a contraction of a muscle. To release it, pull the muscle to lengthen it. You pull in the opposite direction that the cramp is pulling. The following cramp releases work whether you are running, swimming, or lying in bed:

For Calf Cramps:

Calf cramps pull your foot down. To stretch the cramp out, pull your toes up toward the front of your leg and hold. Don't point your foot or start activity again too soon, or the muscle will likely cramp again.

For calf cramps while swimming in shallow water, stop and stand on the noncramping leg and stretch the cramping leg. In deep water, take a big breath and hold it. Float facedown, grasp the offending foot, and do a cramp release while floating. This position makes you resemble a jellyfish with a surface floating body, and arms and legs trailing underwater like tentacles. Remember not to point your foot, or resume the bad kicking that cramped you in the first place. The muscle needs time to settle down.

Figure 30.1. To stop a cramp, stretch the muscle in the opposite direction. To stretch out a calf cramp, pull your foot back and straighten your leg.

For Foot Cramps:

Foot cramps pull your toes down. Grab your toes, pull them back, and hold. While wearing fins, grab the fin tip and pull up and back just as you would for a calf cramp, described above, paying attention to pulling your toes back.

For Hamstring Cramps:

Hamstrings are the triple set of muscles in back of your upper leg. When they contract, whether by choice or by cramp, they bend your knee. To uncramp the hamstrings, straighten your knee and hold.

For Quadriceps Cramps:

Your quadriceps are a set of four muscles (thus the name "quad") in front of your upper leg. When they contract, they straighten your knee. To uncramp the hamstrings, bend your knee and hold.

Other Cramps:

The principles are the same for any spasm your muscles may experience. A common nonleg cramp is a "stitch" in your side, which is a cramp of the diaphragm, your breathing muscle. A "stitch" may occur during a run or other active sport. One way to stretch out a "stitch" is to take a big breath, and hold it while attempting to breath out against the held breath. The pressure stretches things a bit and often releases the cramp. Other people find relief by raising their arms and straightening up, changing from the bent-over position which contracts the muscles.

Back spasms are also common. They can be ruinously painful, frightening, and hindersome to your range of motion and activities. But they are just cramps like all the others and can often be quickly stretched out and relaxed with the proper exercises. They should not be left in spasm for any period of time. Like any other cramp, this makes the muscle more ready to continue the cramp cycle. *See* Chapters 21 and 22 on back and neck pain for more on this.

What About Walking and Pounding?

You may have heard about walking around to stop a leg cramp, or pounding the muscle. These are not very effective, but can work coincidentally. Sometimes people with a calf cramp jump up and walk, which bends back the foot, lengthening the muscle enough to stretch out the spasm. Sometimes the pounding can push a muscle enough to lengthen it, but pounding is likely to make it contract more in sheer defense. Just stretch a cramp, and release the stretch slowly.

Should You Work Through Leg Cramps?

Should you allow a cramp to continue cramping, and just ignore it or keep swimming or whatever you're doing? No. Allowing a muscle to remain in spasm starts a vicious cycle. Spasm itself makes the muscle more "irritable," and ready to cramp again. Just after releasing a cramp, it usually feels like it wants to cramp again. If you point your foot, for example, after a calf cramp and contract the calf muscle again, chances are the calf will cramp again. Beside that, why stay in pain when cramps are so easy to reverse?

How to Prevent Leg Cramps

Daily Habits

Don't walk around all day holding your leg, ankle, and feet muscles tightly. Don't wear tight, uncomfortable shoes, or shoes that you may think are comfortable but that restrict your toes or the natural range of motion of your foot when walking. Take time to exercise, relax, and regularly stretch your legs and feet.

Kick Properly When Swimming

The most effective prevention for leg cramps from kicking while swimming is not to kick with rigid ankles or curled toes. Kicking this way is a bad habit. Many people who kick this way do not know how to kick with loose ankles and floppy feet. The hallmark of people who hold their ankles tightly while kicking in a pool is that they barely make forward progress when using a kickboard without fins on, no matter how hard they kick. Their legs often sink, and kicking is tiring. Don't hold your foot in any one position, and don't deliberately bend it up and down with your kick. Allow it to flop loosely, independent of your leg. This is one of the most important aspects to kicking properly. How can you do that?

Special Exercises

Perhaps you're expecting a list of push-ups, exercises with weights, or running. Here is a surprise. The most important exercise to do if you get leg cramps is a drill to retrain your foot to be completely separate from muscular control while using the rest of your leg:

1. Sit on a chair with your lower legs dangling. At a pool, sit at the rim of the pool, with your lower legs dangling free underwater.
2. Grasp your lower leg near your ankle with both hands. Shake your leg up and down, paying attention to how your foot moves. It should flop freely as you shake it. Don't hold it rigidly angled at the ankle. Don't hook or curl your toes. This may take some work and practice. Let it be as loose and floppy as a rag doll.
3. Carefully observe that as you shake your leg downward, your foot should flop upward, and as you quickly pull your leg up again, your foot flops downward loosely. It should not yank upward as a unit. If you shake side to side, your foot should also swing freely.

Figure 30.2. The floppy foot exercise is important to train your ankle to be loose. Shake your foot, allowing it to flop loosely in whatever direction you shake it.

Doing this exercise until you are successful is crucial for anyone who gets leg cramps while swimming. You can practice this anytime you are sitting comfortably. Someone else can shake your leg, too. Do this until you have retrained your legs' neuromuscular patterns so well that you can flop your feet by quick, small knee movements without using your hands (or someone else's).

The test of a good, loose kick is when you can go into a pool without fins, take a kickboard, and kick with easy forward progress. Most people who have tight ankles make little, sometimes no headway. Those with tight, hooked ankles, who also use a large deep swinging kick, can find themselves traveling backwards. Think of tight ankles, held rigidly at an angle from your leg, as airplane flaps. Trying to move forward with tight ankles is like trying to accelerate with your flaps down. With practice you can loosen your ankles, develop an easy, powerful kick, and eliminate the majority of your leg cramps while swimming.

Leg Stretches

Another useful exercise (although not to be substituted for the floppy-foot drill) is stretching the back of your legs. It's been noted by some muscle-dynamics scientists, that in societies without sit-down toilets, the habitual squatting stretches the appropriate muscles, making calf and foot cramps rare.

No More Leg Cramps

Do regular, easy stretches for your legs and feet, and build up the muscles of your legs so they can handle exertion better. Leg cramps are not something you have to put up with.

31

Funny Physical Facts and Foibles

Laughter is a form of internal jogging. It moves your internal organs around. It enhances respiration. It is an igniter of great expectations.

—Norman Cousins

Why Does It Hurt and Tingle When You Hit Your Funny Bone? Why Do They Call It the Funny Bone? Why Isn't It Funny At All When You Hit It?

It's called the funny bone because it's the humerus.

The humerus is the long bone in your upper arm extending from shoulder to elbow. A nerve called the ulnar nerve runs from your spine through your shoulder through your elbow to your hand. Your ulnar nerve passes closest to your skin's surface just under the knob of bone at the elbow end of your humerus. When you ding your elbow there, you abruptly compress your ulnar nerve against the bone, causing acute temporary pain and numbness.

Your ulnar nerve runs through your elbow in a passageway called the cubital tunnel. In medicine, the word *cubital* refers to the elbow. A person taking your blood pressure will position their stethoscope in the "antecubital space," in front of your elbow. *Cubital* comes from an ancient word that you've probably heard before. If you know the story of Noah's Ark, you remember "cubits," a unit of measure that Noah used to build the Ark. A cubit is the distance from fingertips to elbow. A dinged funny bone is called *transient cubital tunnel syndrome.*

How Much Blood Do You Have To Cut Off Before Your Foot Falls Asleep?

None. The phenomenon of "falling asleep" is not related to blood but to nerve. When you compress a nerve enough, you can temporarily cause the numbing and pins and needles tingling that is popularly called "falling asleep" and medically called neuropraxia (nur-uh-PRAKS-ee-ya). One common, short duration example is banging your funny bone. Sudden compression of the ulnar nerve in your elbow is responsible for the tingling funny bone, as explained above.

Another well-known, longer duration example is the phenomenon occurring in one or both legs after sitting too long at the edge of a bench, particularly in the bathroom. This phenomenon is called "Toilet seat neuropathy" in medical parlance. In this occasion, after sitting too long, you try to stand up but fall over or hop around on tingling feet. The tingling usually quickly reverses.

Where Did the Expression "Knee Jerk Reaction" Come From, and What Does It Really Mean?

You've probably had a physician or someone else tap you just below your kneecap. Your lower leg jumped without your thinking about it. A knee jerk reaction is one you don't think about. In other words, it doesn't use your brain. Here's why: Just below your kneecap is the tendon connecting your four thigh muscles called quadriceps to your lower leg. When the tendon is hit, it stretches slightly but suddenly. The stretched tendon sends a sensory signal, which is a signal about what you felt, up your leg to the part of your spinal cord just above your behind. The signal says, "We're being stretched too fast and it may mean trouble, send help to contract us!" The signal is reflected (that's why it's called a reflex) to a motor nerve. Motor nerves control movement. The motor nerve in your spinal cord sends a signal to your thigh muscles, the quadriceps. The signal says, "Contract!" Your "quads" contract to counter the stretch. Your leg jumps without any input at all from your brain. By the time a separate sensory signal gets all the way up to your brain to tell you that your tendon was stretched, your quads already contracted quickly, making your leg jump. The simple sensory to motor loop that needs no more than your spinal cord to function is called a stretch reflex. You can elicit other stretch reflexes by tapping behind your ankle on your Achilles tendon, or near the crease of your elbow on your biceps tendon.

There are other kinds of reflexes. They vary in complexity but none needs your brain to operate. Sneezing is a reflex reaction to upper respiratory irritation. Coughing is a reflex reaction to lower respiratory irritation. The "wink" reflex closes your eye when something tries to fly in. The "hot stove" reflex yanks your hand away from high heat in the same "sensory-in, motor-out" reaction that, like other reflexes, does not involve conscious thought to initiate action.

Figure 31.1. A knee jerk is a reflex that doesn't use your brain.

The simplest reaction in your body is the reflex, and the "knee jerk" is the simplest of reflexes—only two nerves and no brain.

What Makes You Pumped Up After Lifting Weights? How Does the Muscle Grow That Fast?

Your muscles don't immediately grow in the sense of adding lean weight or splitting muscle fibers. The size increase right after lifting that inflates muscles and egos is only fluid, and temporary fluid at that. When you lift heavy weights, your working muscles contract, compressing the blood vessels in them. Circulation is temporarily reduced or even stopped with extreme muscular contraction.

After you finish lifting weights, a larger volume of blood and fluid than normal rushes back into your muscle, in reaction to the previous deficit. The extra blood puffs up the muscle. There's a fancy technical term for this phenomenon of extra blood puffing up muscles when they react to being contracted. The prefix for an amount greater than normal is *hyper-*. The suffix *-emia,* for blood, comes from the Greek *haima* (from which we get the words *hemorrhage, hemophilia, hemoglobin,* even *hemorrhoid*). Speaking technically, pumping up is called *reactive hyperemia.*

Is It True That If You Put Sleeping People's Hands in a Glass of Water That They Will Wet Themselves?

No. It is not true, but it is always worth a try for the sake of science.

Merely dipping the hand or fingers is ineffective. When you fully immerse your body in water, a real physiologic need to "go" occurs. However, even then, if you are potty-trained, the signals will not override your training. If you were immersed fully during sleep, this would still be so, as long-duration immersion experiments show.

Due to the effects of making you want to go, I have dubbed the increased output occurring with immersion the "P Phenomenon," or PP for short. The "P Phenomenon" happens because immersing your body in water shifts blood away from your arms and legs to the area of your chest called the thorax. Because of buoyancy, fluids just float into the thorax. Being in a cold environment also shifts blood volumes to the thorax. That's why you often notice the "P Phenomenon" when stepping into a cold shower. Volume detectors in the heart notice the increase in fluid and, to normalize thoracic volume, helpfully signal your body to voluntarily show some fluid the way out.

In warm or hot water, however, the phenomenon is reduced. Blood vessels expand in your arms and legs in response to the heat. This peripheral vasodilation shifts blood to your limbs and reduces thoracic blood volume, reducing the physiologic cascade responsible for the P Phenomenon. The fact that warm water reduces the response offers even more evidence against the old glass of water story.

The P Phenomenon even occurs in the microgravity environment of space travel. Fluids float away from the legs and into the upper body, just as during immersion in water. Astronauts have their own technical term for this. They call it "The Fat Face-Chicken-Legs Effect."

What Is the Popping Noise When Your Joints Crack?

Joints pop in several ways. The interesting story starts with bubbles.

A certain amount of nitrogen from the air around you dissolves in your body fluids, including joint fluids called synovial fluids. When pressure is decreased, the gas can come out of its dissolved form. If that happens quickly, bubbles form. There are easy ways for this to happen, for example, popping your knuckles or squatting down and cracking your knees. More on why in a bit. Even scuba divers can do this by coming up from a dive too fast. That does not make noise, but can cause decompression sickness, where bubbles come out of solution in their bodies, get stuck, and cause pain and other problems in all the various places that they get stuck. Then the diver may make a lot of noise. Cracking your knuckles doesn't cause or relate to decompression sickness, although the bubble formation can be similar. Exactly how and why is extraordinarily complex. A summary of a few of the basics follow:

Gases like carbon dioxide and nitrogen are present in dissolved form in your body fluids. They are held in solution by the pressure of air around us and by gas pressures in your body. If you pull your finger joint so that it enlarges briefly, the slight vacuum formed creates a temporary low-pressure cavity. The low pressure pulls gas molecules out of solution forming bubbles in a process called vacuum cavitation. The bubble quickly collapses. Pop. It takes time for the gas to redissolve before the joint can crack again.

Another way bubbles can form besides enlarging the joint space is crushing the muscle against bone, as during some kinds of knuckle and knee cracking. Pop.

Studies have also looked at body tissues (in a laboratory) that are full of dissolved gas (the tissues, not the laboratory). These tissues had no bubbles, even after experimentally subjecting them to large pressure reductions. However, when energy was added by moving the tissue (as happens with muscle contraction) bubbles readily formed. Pop. Pop.

Not all joint cracking is due to bubbles. Often it involves tendons moving quickly over adjacent bony knobs, making a distinctive noise. Pop. Tendons are tough inelastic fibers that connect a muscle to a bone. Snapping tendons occurs routinely in many people's shoulder, elbow, hip, back, and ankle joints. Occasionally tendon snapping occurs in the knee. This kind of snapping, unlike knuckle popping, can be repeated within short intervals, sometimes during every step when walking. Pop. Pop. Pop. Tight muscles can cause that, and specific stretching exercises can relieve it. On rare occasions it is so painful, constant, and detrimental to sports activity that surgery is performed to move the tendon to a slightly different position to avoid the snapping.

Another reason for joint popping can come from bad sitting, standing, and lifting postures all day. As muscles tighten and contract unevenly, tendons or ligaments can get pulled slightly away from their accustomed track. People often learn that they can "crack" their back to restore a more comfortable position. Pop. Although it often feels good, it is not a miracle cure. It is better to learn to identify and minimize the muscle stress that caused the need in the first place.

How detrimental knuckle and other joint cracking may be to your joints depends on degree. It's probably safe to avoid any vigorous trauma to your joints. Joints are important parts of your body. Joint deterioration is related to the extent of abuse, genetics, and other not-well-identified factors. Although not a certainty, chronic, traumatic joint stress may be a contributor to early wear and tear that may lead to arthritic degeneration.

Not All "Knuckle" Popping Is in Your Body

Marine propellers cavitate bubbles by similar mechanical forces as knuckle popping. The rotating propeller blade rapidly forms low-pressure areas. Dissolved gas cavitates out of the water near the blades. When these many tiny bubbles suddenly form then collapse with great vigor against the blade, they make noise and eventually pit the blade. Pop. Pop. Pop. Anticavitation devices are important tools to extend the life of propellers and minimize military submarine noise.

Why Does Hair Grow Back Thicker and/or Darker When You Shave It?

It doesn't. This old tale is hard to kill. There is a reason hair seems to change, when it really doesn't. All body hair is thicker, and usually darker, at the base than tip. When you shave, you cut off the thinner, lighter tips. When the rest of the hair shaft starts growing past the skin line again, you see only the thicker, darker part of the hair you cut. When that decapitated hair finally reaches the end of its cycle and falls out, the hair growing to replace it is not altered from its original shape or genetically determined color. If you shave again before this happens, you will feel the stubby growth again soon enough.

As far as boys shaving for the first time, the beard typically becomes coarser with the passing years of manhood, whether shaved or not. Hair change with maturation should not be confused for effects of shaving.

Why Are the Areas on the Side of the Head Called Temples?

The word *temple* comes from the Greek word for "time." The sides of the face near the ears are usually the first to go gray, evidencing the inevitable passage of time.

Figure 31.2. Football players do not play better by breathing supplemental oxygen.

Does Oxygen Make You Feel Good?

Breathing oxygen is popularly thought to help football players, make you feel good, cure headaches, and work wildly as an aphrodisiac. All these claims have been firmly disproven—except one.

Chapter 4, "What Does 'Aerobic' Really Mean?," explained that breathing oxygen will not help football players. The sprints and tackles in football are so short that the body fuel that is used is quick and ready stored fuel, not oxygen. Football may be a hard sport, but it is not an aerobic one.

Studies by the Department of Internal Medicine at Baylor University, and reported in the *Journal of the American Medical Association,* found no advantage to breathing 100% oxygen on recovery from exhaustive bouts of exercise, no difference in performance during a second bout after breathing 100% oxygen, and that the professional athletes who served as subjects could not identify whether they were breathing 100% oxygen or room air. In other studies, a percentage of subjects who were told they were breathing oxygen but received room air reported elevated mood.

Breathing supplemental oxygen benefits exercise if breathed *during* long duration, heavy exercise. Heart rate and blood levels of lactic acid decrease, and time to exhaustion increases. Still, carrying oxygen tanks while jogging or biking presents interesting practical problems. If you want to get more oxygen to your cells for greater long-distance ability there is another way to do it yourself. Regular aerobic training enhances your body's entire oxygen carrying and using system.

As for effect on libido, there is no evidence of any physical aphrodisiac capability of oxygen. The placebo effect is potent in this area.

It is in relieving cluster headaches that oxygen seems to work. Breathing 100% oxygen constricts brain blood vessels. One of the mechanisms proposed for at least one stage of cluster headache is enlarged brain blood vessels that inflame and hurt. Oxygen is under study as a treatment for cluster headache (more on this in Chapter 29, "Headaches").

Oxygen is a good invention, no doubt. Many purported properties are fiction. But some are real. You can feel good about that.

Glossary

A

Acetabulum [From Latin *acetum,* "vinegar," from which we get acetic acid. Acetabulum is a shallow vinegar vessel or cup.] Cup-shaped hollow in the hipbones, where the head of the upper leg bone (femur) fits. The socket of the ball and socket joint. The acetabulum is located at the junction of the three hipbones, the ilium, ischium, and pubis bone. *See* Femur, Ilium, Ischium, and Pubis.

Acromion [From Greek *akros,* "extreme," or "tip" + *omion,* diminutive of *omos,* "shoulder."] The bone of the outer end of your shoulder, formed by the shoulder blade (scapula) winging around to the front of the shoulder. Your collarbone attaches in front.

Adenosine Triphosphate (ATP) (un-DEN-oh-sintry-FOS-fate) [Named for its adenosine base plus three phosphates.] The molecule made in your body that supplies energy to your cells for all your biochemical processes. It has two phosphates held on by low-energy bonds, and a third with a high-energy bond. ATP releases energy by breaking off the phosphate with the high-energy bond, becoming adenosine *di*phosphate (ADP). In extreme situations, ADP loses another phosphate to become adenosine monophosphate (AMP), but little more energy is gained as that is a low-energy bond. You have three systems that make ATP—one is aerobic and two are *an*aerobic. *See* Aerobic Metabolism, Anaerobic Metabolism, and Creatine Phosphate (CP).

Aerobic Capacity   *See* Endurance, Cardiovascular.

Aerobic Exercise   Activities that are long and intense enough to benefit your cardiovascular system, but not so intense that your *an*aerobic energy-making systems have to do much work. Just sitting in a chair uses your aerobic metabolism for about 100% of your energy needs, but it is not an aerobic exercise. Sprinting down the street at top speed is exercise, but is so high intensity that your anaerobic systems predominate: your aerobic system can't supply energy fast enough. Jogging or swimming or bicycling for 20 minutes or longer at a pace where you are not greatly out of breath is aerobic exercise.

Aerobic Metabolism   System of making ATP (an energy molecule) using oxygen with stored carbohydrate, fat, and protein. Aerobic metabolism goes on all day and night, even when you're sitting around or sleeping, making a distinction between aerobic metabolism and aerobic exercise. In animals it takes place in the cells' organelles called mitochondria. Your aerobic system has two pathways, the Krebs cycle and the electron transport chain. You make most of your ATP in the electron transport chain. When you exercise aerobically, oxygen carries off hydrogen ions transforming lactic acid back to pyruvate, which can be used to make ATP. It also means that lactic acid does not get a chance to build up as it does when you are anaerobic. Your aerobic system allows you to generate energy for long, low- to moderate-intensity activities. Your aerobic metabolism can supply much energy, but can't do it very fast. Your *an*aerobic systems allow you to do quick, high-intensity activities. The combination of systems makes your exercise capacity very versatile. *See* Adenosine Triphosphate (ATP), Anaerobic Metabolism, Electron Transport Chain, and Krebs Cycle,

Aldosterone   (al-DOHS-tur-own) [Named for its chemical structure containing an aldehyde and a sterol.] Steroid hormone secreted by the adrenal gland and regulated by the kidney. Helps you retain salt and water, and excrete potassium, to maintain their healthy balance in your body.

Allergy   [From Greek *allos,* "other" + *ergon,* "action."] Condition where a person may react with sneezing, itching, and skin rashes to things like pollen, foods, or microorganisms, which cause no reaction in other people. Term coined by Austrian physician Pirquet, around the early 1900s.

Amenorrhea (ay-men-or-REE-ah) [*a-*, "without" + Greek *men*, "month".] Long-term cessation of menstruation due to several causes, most notably low estrogen. A risk factor for osteoporosis.

Amphetamines [Composite word from A(lpha) + M(ethyl) + PH(enyl) + ET(hyl) + amine.] A group of stimulant drugs, sometimes used to increase athletic performance, to reduce fatigue, or reduce hunger as an ingredient in diet pills. They are sympathomimetic, as they mimic the activation of your sympathetic nervous system, primarily by releasing nerve transmission chemicals called catecholamines, especially epinephrine (adrenaline) and norepinephrine (noradrenaline) from nerve endings. *See* Catecholamine, Ergogenic Aid, Sympathetic Nervous System, and Sympathomimetic.

Anabolic Steroids Drugs capable of increasing muscle growth. Not all steroids are anabolic, for example, the antiinflammatories prednisone and cortisone, and Vitamin D. Since anabolic steroids have many dangerous effects along with their muscle-building ones, they are prescription substances. Bodybuilders sometimes try to find non-regulated sources. There are no true anabolic steroids sold in health food stores, although many products that are just regular food have labels suggesting that they have anabolic effects. This is not illegal. The consumer needs to become educated to watch out for such misleading claims. *See* Ergogenic Aid.

Anaerobic Capacity Ability of your body to use special stored fuel, not oxygen, for rapid-onset, short-duration, intense activity. Because it is not an oxygen-using (aerobic) system, it is called *an*aerobic. You use your anaerobic system for sprinting, swimming against hard currents, lifting heavy weights, and any short, intense activity. You can improve your anaerobic capacity by exercising anaerobically, that is, practicing short, intense exercises. *See* Anaerobic Metabolism, and compare to Aerobic Exercise and Aerobic Metabolism.

Anaerobic Metabolism Two systems of making ATP, a special energy molecule, without using any oxygen. The first system is your ATP-CP system of stored ATP. The second anaerobic system is glycolysis. It is important for you to have systems of making energy without using oxygen for the many activities that begin so quickly, and are so high intensity, that your oxygen system is not able to supply your needs. Your anaerobic systems allow you to do quick, high-intensity activities. Anaerobic metabolism can't make much ATP, but can do it very quickly. Your aerobic system allows you to generate energy for long, low- to moderate-intensity activities. The combination of systems makes your exercise capacity very versatile. *See* Adenosine Triphosphate (ATP), Aerobic Metabolism, and Glycolysis.

Anorexia Nervosa [From Greek *an,* "without" + *orexis,* "appetite" (from *oregein,* "to reach out for.")] An abnormal loss of appetite and refusal to eat resulting in emaciation and malnutrition. A risk factor for osteoporosis.

Anthropometrics (an-throw-poh-MET-tricks) [From Greek *anthrapos,* "human being" + *metrikos,* from *metron,* "measure."] Science of identifying and comparing human body measurements, such as lengths and widths of segments, to those of other segments, and to those of other people. One use of anthropometrics is to measure bone lengths and widths at specific joints to tell the size of your body's frame—small, medium, or large—which helps determine optimum weight. Another use of anthropometrics is to predict the sport you might excel in, based on your specific body size and other anthropometric measurements.

Antihistamine [From Greek *anti,* "opposite" + histamine.] An agent that reduces the effects of an inflammatory chemical called histamine. Both histamines and antihistamines are naturally produced in your body, but you occasionally need a "boost" of an oral or injectable antihistamine. Antihistamines work by blocking or displacing histamine at its sites of action. *See* Histamine.

Apnea (AP-nee-uh) [From Greek *a-,* "without" + *pnoia,* "breathing."] Temporary halt to breathing. Examples are voluntary breath holding while swimming underwater, and involuntary lapses from sleep disorders involving snoring. *See* Sleep Apnea.

Apples and Pears Body classification system to predict, in a very general way, a tendency toward cardiovascular risk and obesity-linked disease. People who store fat primarily in the upper body and abdomen have bodies that resemble an apple shape, while pear-shaped people store fat mostly around the hips and thighs. Apple shape is associated with higher disease risk than pear shape.

Arrhythmia [From Greek *a,* "without" + *ruthmia,* "rhythm."] Irregular heartbeat. Arrhythmias occur normally now and then among normal heartbeats, without ill effect or your being aware of them. Too many arrhythmias, occurring too often, can be harmful.

Arteries Muscular, elastic, branching system of thick-walled tubes carrying blood away from the heart to all the body. *See* Veins.

Arthritis [From Greek *arthron,* "joint," + *itis,* inflammation.] Inflammation of a joint, or joints, with pain, swelling, loss of function, and sometimes deformity of the joint. There are different kinds of arthritis. Degenerative, or osteoarthritis, involves wearing away the smooth cartilage on bone ends (articular cartilage). Osteoarthritis can be because of, or along with, trauma to the joint or other conditions. Other kinds of arthritis, like rheumatoid arthritis, are due to an autoimmune attack by the body against itself. Arthritis is treated with antiinflammatory medications and exercise.

Atherosclerotic Plaques   [From Greek *athero,* "gruel-like," + *sclerosis,* "hardening."] Irregular deposits of lipid in the lining of medium and large arteries. Associated with cardiovascular disease.

B

Ball and Socket Joint   Type of joint, found in the shoulder and hip, allowing rotary motion in every direction through the movement of the ball in the socket. The ball part is a roundish knob of one bone that fits into a cavity or socket of the other. Also called enarthrosis. *See* Acetabulum and Femoral Neck.

Body Mass Index   (BMI). Pen and paper test for obesity, obtained by taking your weight in kilograms divided by height in meters squared. If BMI is above 25, you are considered by this test to be fat. If over 30, you are considered obese.

Bones   Semistiff connective tissue that holds up all your other soft squishy parts. Bones in various parts of your body have varying amounts of a dense, compact, outer layer, called cortical bone, and an inner loose, spongy trabecular bone. The central part of a long bone is filled with marrow. Bones are covered by the periosteum. Bones are not all hard inorganic mineral. Bone is about 75% inorganic material and 25% organic material. The protein, or collagen portion of bones gives them flexibility and resiliency. If you remove the calcium from a bone by soaking it in vinegar, the bone would become as flexible as a dog's rubber plaything-bone. *See* Cortical Bone, Periosteum, and Trabecular Bone.

Bradycardia   [From Greek *brady,* "slow" + *kardia,* "heart."] Slow heart rate in an adult human, usually fewer than 60 beats per minute.

Bronchi   (BRON-kai) [From Greek *bronkhos,* "windpipe."] Plural of bronchus. The two branches of your windpipe leading to your lungs.

Bursa   [From Greek, "wineskin," "purse."] A little sac containing viscous lubricating fluid, located where a tendon passes over a bone, or at points of friction between moving body structures. You have over 70 bursas in many places in your body. Chronically irritating a bursa can result in inflammation, called bursitis. Shoulder bursitis can result from bad shoulder exercises. Knee bursitis can result from too much kneeling (what used to be called housemaid's knee).

C

Cadaver Analysis Body fat determination technique of cutting the body open to directly measure fat stores.

Calcium Balance The amount of body calcium gain versus loss. Positive calcium balance occurs when more calcium is absorbed from the diet than excreted. The excess can deposit in the skeleton. When loss exceeds absorption, calcium will mobilize (be taken) from bone, a process called negative calcium balance. Eating more calcium will not automatically deposit that calcium in your bones.

Calipers [Alteration of caliber.] Small instrument used for measuring diameters. Calipers used for body composition analysis measure the thickness of your folds of fat. Caliper measurement is painless, except by overenthusiastic testers. The error of measurement can often be large, varying greatly with tester experience. Calipers are often misused in health clubs. If, for example, you are measured at 25% the first time, and 22% the second time, it is incorrect to state that you lost 3% fat. Because of the error of measurement, that is impossible to tell.

Carbohydrate [From Latin *carbon* + Greek *hudro,* "water," because they are made of carbon, hydrogen, and oxygen.] Organic compounds including sugar, starch, and cellulose. Found in nutritional quantities only in plants, they are a major energy source for many animals, including humans. Animals store a carbohydrate called glycogen in their muscles and liver, but not enough to supply any appreciable amount if the animal is eaten. For that reason, meat is not considered to have any carbohydrate. *See* Glycogen.

Carbohydrate Loader Drink Beverage containing carbohydrate, used to replace fluids and delay fatigue in long endurance events. *See* Carbohydrate, Carbohydrate Replacer Drink, and Electrolyte.

Carbohydrate Replacer Drink High-carbohydrate beverage, used both to replace fluids and restock your body's carbohydrate supply after long endurance events. *See* Carbohydrate, Carbohydrate Loader Drink, and Electrolyte.

Catecholamine (cat-eh-COAL-uh-meen) [Named for its chemical structure derived from a catechol and an amine.] Important family of nervous system chemicals that work as both neurotransmitters and hormones to transmit signals in your body. Some of your important catecholamines are dopamine, norepinephrine, and epinephrine. Your body makes them in sequential steps, starting with the amino acid tyrosine. Each step turns each catecholamine into the next. First you make tyrosine into DOPA. From DOPA you make dopamine.

From dopamine you make norepinephrine. From norepinephrine you make epinephrine (same as adrenaline).

Cervical Vertebrae [From Latin *cervic,* "neck."] The seven bones of your neck. They are named sequentially down from your head as C1–C7. If you tip your head forward and feel the back of your neck, the most prominent bump is your C7 vertebra. Your other six cervical vertebrae are above it. Below C7 begin your 12 thoracic vertebrae, which are the bones of your upper back. *See* Thoracic Vertebrae, Lumbar Vertebrae, and Vertebra.

Cholesterol [From Greek *khole,* "bile" (because it was first found in gallstones) and from which we get words like gall and gold, + Greek *stereos,* "solid."] Made in your liver, cholesterol is an important constituent of all your cell membranes, and a precursor to steroid hormones. Also influences development of cardiovascular disease. Cholesterol circulates in your blood plasma, carried around by proteins of various densities (lipoproteins). Cholesterol is the most abundant steroid in animal tissues, but not found at all in plants. *See* High-Density Lipoprotein Cholesterol, and Low-Density Lipoprotein Cholesterol.

Claudication [From Latin *claudico,* "to limp."] Leg pain from clogged blood vessels in the legs.

Coccyx (KOKS-icks) [G. *kokkyx,* "cuckoo," from its resemblance to a cuckoo's beak.] Tail bone. The small triangular bone at the end of the spine in human beings and tailless apes. Made of four fused rudimentary vertebrae. *See* Cervical Vertebrae, Thoracic Vertebrae, Lumbar Vertebrae, and Vertebra.

Coca Leaves [Coca is Spanish, from the Quechua *kúka.*] Dried leaves of certain small shrubs or trees, genus Erythroxylum, especially E. coca. The leaves contain cocaine and other alkaloids, and are chewed for a stimulating effect by people of the Andes to help tolerate hunger, fatigue, and altitude, or harvested and purified for making cocaine. *See* Ergogenic Aid.

Coenzyme A body chemical that you need to enhance or promote the action of an enzyme. Coenzymes are smaller than the enzymes they work with. Usually contains a vitamin or mineral combined with a specific protein. Sometimes coenzymes are misrepresented as able to improve physical ability if taken orally, which is not the case. Like all proteins, they are broken down in to component parts to digest and pass through the intestinal wall. They will not automatically reassemble into the original coenzyme on the other side. *See* Enzyme and Ergogenic Aid.

Cortical Bone [From Latin *cortex,* "bark."] Also called compact bone.

Dense, strong bone forming the outside shell or wall of your long bones. When bone loss occurs with normal (and accelerated) aging processes, cortical bone loss occurs later than trabecular bone loss. *See* Bone, Periosteum, and Trabecular Bone.

Cramp [Possibly from Middle Dutch *crampe,* "hook" to restrict or prevent from free action or expression.] Sudden, involuntary, painful muscle spasm, or shortening. Stretching the muscle to lengthen it releases the cramp. Cramp releases can be easily done yourself on leg, foot, and side cramps, and for back spasms yourself or by orthopedists, osteopaths, and trained massage therapists and physical therapists.

Creatine Phosphate (CP) [Named for its composition of creatine with phosphoric acid.] Organic compound in your muscles that stores and provides energy for muscular contraction. Breaking down creatine phosphate provides the phosphate you need to make ATP, the bottom-line energy molecule for all your body processes. Also called phosphocreatine. *See* Adenosine Triphosphate (ATP).

D

Disc [From Greek *diskos,* "to throw."] Round, flat, fibrocartilage cushion between certain bones. You have tiny little discs between your jawbone (mandible) and your head bone (temporal bone). Sometimes these discs wear out causing pain at the joint between those two bones called the temporomandibular joint (TMJ), causing TMJ pain. Your vertebral discs lie between the bones of your spine (vertebrae). Vertebral discs are commonly injured over time by bad sitting, standing, and lifting postures, particularly the discs of the lower back (lumbar vertebrae). That is where people most commonly load the greatest stresses through bad lifting, sitting, and standing habits. *See* Disc Herniation and Lumbar Vertebrae.

Disc Herniation (slipped discs) Protrusion of a vertebral disc beyond its normal place. Can cause pain by itself, and also by pressing on nerves and other structures, which causes pain away from the site of the herniation. Disc herniations are easily caused over time by bad sitting, standing, and lifting habits, and usually easily treated without surgery, by good back habits and exercises.

Dorsiflex [From Latin *dorsum,* "back" + flex, "to bend."] Turning the hand or foot toward the upper side. To bend at the ankle so that the toes point backward toward the top of the foot. *See* Plantarflex.

Dowager's Hump Curved hunched appearance of the upper back in both men and women, caused by osteoporotic crush fractures of the thoracic vertebrae (bones of the upper back). *See* Osteoporosis.

E

Electrolyte [From Greek *electro* + *lytos* and *lysis,* "soluble" or "loosening," from which we get words such as *dialysis, electrolysis,* and *analysis.*] Any substance which, when dissolved in a liquid, becomes electrically conductive, because it breaks up into ions. Ions are atoms or molecules with at least one electron more or less than normal for it, giving it a negative or positive charge. For example, table salt (sodium chloride) breaks down in water into the positive sodium ion and the negative chloride ion. In physiology, the term *electrolyte* usually refers to the ions, rather than the original substance. Your cells use electrolytes to regulate processes such as flow of water across the cell membrane. Ions propagate signals along nerves for all the thousands of functions that nerves control to keep you alive, moving, and thinking. Two of your principal positively charged ions (electrolytes) are sodium and potassium. Magnesium and calcium are also positive ions. Two important negatively charged ions are chloride and bicarbonate.

Electrolyte Drink Beverage containing electrolytes and, usually, carbohydrates to supply water, electrolytes, and carbohydrate before, during, or after exercise.

Electron Transport Chain A sequence of reactions that are part of how you make ATP energy aerobically. Electrons from the Krebs cycle get transported to oxygen by little electron carriers. The electrons pass through a series of iron-containing proteins called cytochromes (close relatives of hemoglobin). Each player in the series is increasingly fond of electrons, so that the entire series runs "downhill," and energy is produced. Energy not used for chemical work dissipates as heat. The electron transport chain is also called the respiratory chain and the cytochrome system. *See* Adenine Triphosphate and Krebs cycle.

Endorphin [Composite word from *endogenous* ("made from within") + "morphine-like substance".] A class of hormones produced by a number of processes, including extended, hard exercise. Not confirmed, but along with other opioid chemicals produced in the body, possibly associated with positive mood after good workouts.

Endurance, Cardiovascular [From Latin *indurare,* "to harden".] Ability of your heart and lungs to get oxygen and nutrients to your body for fuel during exercise. Determines duration you can continue at a given pace. Needed for continuous, mid- and low-intensity walking, running, skiing, swimming, cycling, etc. Also called cardiorespiratory endurance, aerobic capacity, or functional capacity. *See* Aerobic Metabolism, Anaerobic Capacity, and Anaerobic Metabolism.

Endurance, Muscular Ability of muscles to move a relatively light weight repeatedly. Walking, swimming, finning, cycling, running, even sitting and standing up straight all day require muscular endurance.

Enzyme [From Greek *en-,* "in" + *zume,* yeast, from which we get the word *zymurgy,* the branch of chemistry dealing with fermenting and brewing alcohol. From the Greek word *zein,* "to boil."] A protein which speeds up chemical reactions. Enzymes function by holding other molecules in just the right way so that they can put together the molecules or break them apart. Examples of enzymes that help break apart other molecules are lactase, which breaks down lactose in milk; amylase in your saliva, which starts breaking down carbohydrates you eat; papain, a plant enzyme used in meat tenderizer that breaks down meat protein; and zymase, the enzyme in yeast that breaks down sugar into alcohol and carbon dioxide. The various synthetase enzymes help put molecules together. With notable exceptions, names of most enzymes end in the suffix *-ase.* All enzymes are proteins. Enzymes that you eat are destroyed by digestion before they can pass into your bloodstream and reach your body tissues. Digesting means breaking down to components small enough to pass through the intestinal wall. It will not automatically reassemble into the original enzyme on the other side of the intestinal wall. Eating enzymes, even those promoted as health foods (except digestive aids), will not raise body enzyme levels. *See* Coenzyme.

Ergogenic Aid [From Greek *ergon,* "work" + *gen,* "producing" or "generating".] Products that enhance physical ability. Ergogenic aids may be nutritional, psychological, or physical. Not everything claimed to be ergogenic is ergogenic. There are many sham products on the market. Some ergogenic aids do work, such as weight lifting, caffeine, and amphetamines. Not all dietary products sold as ergogenic aids are completely healthful or non-habit-forming, such as the several stimulant herbs on the market, or products containing caffeine. *See* Amphetamines, Anabolic Steroids, Coenzyme, Ginseng, Ma huang, Minerals, and Vitamins.

Extension Increasing the angle of a joint. Elbow extension is straightening a bent arm. Knee extension is straightening the knee. Neck and back extension involve moving your head or torso, respectively,

away from a bent forward position. Hyperextension is extending
the joint past a straight line, or 180 degrees. *See* Flexion.

F

Facets, Vertebral   [From Old French *facette,* "little face."] Small, smooth
areas on your spine bones (vertebrae), where one vertebra fits
together with the next. If injured over time with bad back posture,
they can be a cause of back pain. Usually associated with chronic,
excessive, arching postures.

Fat   A greasy substance found in the adipose tissue of animals, and in
the seeds and nuts of plants. In animals, fat is the principal storage
form for energy. As a food, fat gives you 9 calories per gram. Carbohydrate and protein, by comparison, give you 4 calories per gram. *See*
Carbohydrate and Protein.

Femoral Neck   Slender part of your upper thigh bone (femur) between
the long bone of your femur and the "ball" part of your femur, called
the femoral head. The femoral head fits into the "socket" of your
hip, called the acetabulum. The femoral neck is a common site of
osteoporotic fracture. *See* Acetabulum, Ball and Socket Joint, Femur.

Femur   [From Latin for thigh.] Thighbone. Upper leg bone, between
your hip and knee. It is the largest and strongest bone in your body.

Flexibility   [From Latin *flexibilis,* "to bend."] Ability to move safely and
comfortably through a range of motion required to do the things
you want to do.

Flexion   [From Latin *flectere,* "to bend."] Decreasing the angle of a
joint. Elbow flexion, for example, is bending your arm. Knee flexion
involves bending the knee. (*Genu* is the Latin word for "knee,"
giving us the word *genuflection.*) Neck and back flexion involve
curling your head or torso, respectively, toward a bent forward
position. Too much flexion in your lower back, usually from poor
posture when sitting, contributes to back pain. *See* Extension.

Folic Acid   [From Latin *folium,* "leaf," for its common occurrence in
leafy vegetables.] Substance from the Vitamin B complex group,
occurring in green plants, fresh fruit, and yeast. Also called folacin,
folate, and Vitamin BC. Deficiency of folic acid is known to be
associated with birth defects, and more recently with heart disease
and stroke. Eating more green leafy vegetables adds folic acid to
your diet.

Food Pyramid   A schematic of seven food groups needed for nutritional
health. The food pyramid replaces old "four food groups." Large
helpings of fruits, grains, and vegetables form the large, solid base

of the pyramid. Small groups at the top of the pyramid include a protein group that includes beans and meat, and an even smaller sugar and fat group to eat sparingly. Food pyramid recommendations agree on vegetables as main dishes, with meat as side dishes if you eat meat, not the other way around.

Four Food Groups   A now obsolete system of grouping foods into four categories to be eaten at every meal. It has been found that diets based on the four categories were high fat, and had only about half of the minimum daily required amounts of needed nutrients.

Free Radical   An atom, molecule, or macromolecule existing temporarily with at least one unpaired electron. Electrons usually prefer to be paired. Being unpaired makes them reactive and eager either to acquire another electron or to lose the unpaired one. Some free radicals are beneficial, such as those involved in muscle contraction and in the immune response, while others are detrimental, such as those involved in certain disease processes and oxygen toxicity. Free radicals occur normally as a by-product of breathing, and in increased numbers during exercise, in smog, from cigarette smoke, and in high-pressure oxygen environments. In 1954, Rebecca Gershman and her colleagues, in a theory now widely accepted, proposed that the damaging effects of oxygen toxicity are caused by oxygen free radicals. An oxygen free radical has one unpaired electron. It strongly wants to take an electron from other molecules, particularly fatty acids and proteins. When oxygen free radicals grab electrons from hemoglobin, cell membranes, or protein enzymes, those substances are rendered ineffective at their former jobs. In addition, they become free radicals themselves, with a strong propensity to grab electrons from others, starting a chain of destructive events (like a game of tag). The body produces various antioxidant substances to neutralize many free radicals.

G

Gastrocnemius   [From Greek *gastro,* "belly," referring to the largest part of a muscle + *kneme,* "leg."] Large, prominent muscle of the calf of your leg. Attaches to your Achilles tendon and pulls on the tendon to pull your foot downward (plantarflex).

Ginseng   [From Mandarin Chinese *ren,* "person" + *shen,* collective name of a variety of herbs with fat, fleshy roots sometimes resembling the human body.] Any of several plants, or roots of plants of genus *Panax,* particularly *P. pseudoginseng,* of eastern Asia, or *P. quinque-*

folius of North America. Stimulates your nervous system, raising heart rate and blood pressure. *See* Ergogenic Aid.

Glycogen [From Greek, *glukos,* "sweet" + *gen,* "making" or "producing."] The form that glucose (sugar) is stored in your body, mostly in your liver and muscles. Glycogen is converted to glucose through a series of enzymatic steps, to meet your body's rapid energy needs. *See* Glycolysis.

Glycogen Loading An exercise and diet procedure to increase the amount of glycogen you can store. Greater stores of glycogen extend your exercise capacity.

Glycogen Sparing Body process of using more fat as an exercise fuel, and less glycogen, and so "sparing" the glycogen. Glycogen sparing allows more time until your glycogen stores are exhausted, allowing you to exercise longer. Being in better shape "teaches" your body better glycogen sparing.

Glycolysis [From Greek *glukos,* "sweet" + *lysis,* "breaking down" or "loosening," seen in words such as *dialysis, electrolysis,* and *analysis.*] Metabolic process of breaking down carbohydrates and sugars, typically glucose, to generate ATP, your "bottom-line" energy molecule. Occurs in almost all living cells. In humans, the last product generated by glycolysis while making ATP aerobically is pyruvic acid (anaerobic glycolysis). When you are anaerobic, the process goes one more step to lactic acid (anaerobic glycolysis). When you have enough oxygen, the lactic acid can be changed back to pyruvic acid. This series of reactions was described by Gustav Embden and Otto Meyerhof in the 1930s, and so is sometimes called the Embden-Meyerhof cycle. Glycolysis can make only two molecules of ATP from a molecule of glucose, while your aerobic metabolism can make 36. Being aerobic makes more energy, which is why your aerobic system lets you exercise longer than your anaerobic system. *See* Adenisin Triphospate, Glycogen, Lactic Acid, and Pyruvic Acid.

H

Hamstring Muscles The triple set of muscles of the back of your upper leg. Your hamstring muscles work to bend your knee and straighten your hip. Your two innermost hamstrings, or medial hamstrings, are the semimembranosus and the semitendinosus muscles. Your outside, or lateral hamstring, is the biceps femoris muscle. The term *hamstrings* is also used to refer to the tendons of the three muscles, readily felt as stringy cords on either side of the hollow of the back of your knee.

Hemochromatosis [Greek *haima,* "blood" + *khroma,* "color" + *osis,* "condition."] A hereditary disorder of iron metabolism, where you absorb and keep too much of the iron you eat. The iron deposits in the tissues, particularly the liver, pancreas, and skin, where it causes a bronze coloration and constant fatigue. Eventually, heart and liver failure may occur.

High-Density Lipoprotein Cholesterol Popularly called "good cholesterol." Compound containing lipid (fat) and protein. HDL removes cholesterol from your bloodstream, and does not collect on or stick to the inner linings of your arteries. You can increase your levels of HDL with exercise and low-fat meals. *See* Cholesterol and Low-Density Lipoprotein Cholesterol.

Hip Flexors Muscles that bend (flex) your hip into a sitting position. Many people confuse hip flexor exercises that bend the hip, like sit-ups and leg lifts, for abdominal exercises that, properly done, would involve only the abdominal muscles that curl the trunk. The three major hip flexors are the iliacus, psoas (SEW-as), and rectus femoris. The iliacus and psoas, often lumped together as the iliopsoas, are the "filet mignon" muscles. Beef animals are prevented from exercising their hip flexors to make the muscle soft and fatty for humans to eat. Tight hip flexor muscles contribute to poor posture, back pain, and surprisingly, shoulder injuries, when the shoulder has to overrotate to reach overhead when tight hip flexors do not allow full range of motion of your torso.

Histamine [Named because it is an amine derived from histidine, and so hist (idine) + amine.] An amine released from cells of your immune system as part of an allergic reaction. Histamine powerfully stimulates gastric secretions, constricts bronchial smooth muscle which restricts breathing, and dilates small blood vessels. Sometimes this dilation is extensive enough to cause a drop in blood pressure. *See* Antihistamine.

Homeostasis [From Greek *homos,* "same" + *stasis,* "standstill."] Continuous regulation of all the body's goings-on, using physiologic checks and balances to maintain the system at its set equilibrium. Body temperature, oxygen levels, pH, water balance, plasma ion regulation, calorie utilization, and many other processes are all tightly regulated. The principle was first described by French physiologist Claude Bernard, and later given its name by Walter Cannon, a Harvard physiologist,

Homeotherm (HOME-ee-oh-thurms) [From Greek *homos,* "same" + *therme,* "heat."] Animals who generate and regulate heat internally to maintain a largely constant body temperature that is independent of, and typically above, surrounding temperature. Birds and mammals are homeotherms. Sometimes called endotherms. *See* Poikilotherm.

Hormone   [From Greek *horman,* "to urge on."] Chemical messengers, usually peptides or steroids, produced in one body tissue and traveling through your blood to stimulate or suppress activity in another tissue. Examples, among many, are insulin, adrenaline (epinephrine), and antidiuretic hormone (ADH). Hormones regulate body processes as diverse as growth, metabolism, reproduction, and modification of behavior.

Hydrostatic Weighing   Also called underwater weighing. Body composition analysis technique to determine body fat, called the "gold standard" because it has a very low error of measurement, and other tests of body composition are often compared in percentage error to hydrostatic weighing. To be weighed hydrostatically, you sit on a scale in a vat of water, then exhale all you can while keeping your entire body underwater.

Hypertonic   [Prefix *hyper,* "more" or "above"+ Greek *tonos,* "tension."] In chemistry, a solution containing a higher concentration of dissolved particles compared to a reference solution, usually blood or body tissues. For example, sea water is hypertonic to your blood (about three times more concentrated). *See* Hypotonic and Isotonic.

Hypotonic   [hypo, "less" or "under" + Greek *tonos,* "tension."] In chemistry, a solution containing a smaller concentration of dissolved particles compared to a reference solution, usually blood or body tissues. For example, fresh water is hypotonic to your blood. *See* Hypertonic and Isotonic.

Hypovolemic Thirst   One of your two thirst mechanisms. Stimulated by low body water stores. *See* Osmotic Thirst.

Hypoxia   [Prefix *hypo* + *oxia,*"oxygen."] Condition in which insufficient oxygen reaches body tissues. Distinct from (but usually related to) hypoxemia, which is insufficient oxygenation of blood.

I

Ilium   [From Latin *ilium,* "groin" or "flank."] The widest and uppermost of the three bones that make up each side of your pelvis. The ilium on each side of your hips can be felt as the "shelf" that you can rest a bundle on. *See* Ischium and Pubis (your other two pelvic bones).

Inflammation   [From Latin, *in* + *flammare,* "to set on fire."] Response of body tissues to an injury, bite, sting, or infection. Characterized by warmth (calor), redness (rubor), swelling (tumor), and pain (dolor). Inflammation attracts immune cells, which secrete free radicals to kill bacteria and other invaders. *See* Free Radical.

Insensible Perspiration   Sweat that evaporates before you are aware of it. The term sometimes includes evaporation from your respiratory tract.

Insulinogenic   [Insulin + Greek *gen,* "producing."] Substance that encourages insulin production. Sometimes carbohydrate products are misrepresented in health food stores as special foods that stimulate insulin. Because one function of insulin is to encourage protein storage, advertisers lead people to believe that eating such food will build muscle. But just about any food is insulinogenic, and another function of insulin is to aid fat storage. Conversely, a popular high-protein diet promotes the idea that you must avoid nonprotein foods because they stimulate insulin, leading to more fat storage, and eat only high-protein foods. That also seems to be misleading (and potentially unhealthy). The high-protein diets "work" because they are low-calorie, not for any insulin-stimulating or -suppressing quality.

Insurance Tables   Predetermined values in insurance company tables of ranges of "acceptable" weights for various heights and frame sizes. Usually, if you are more than 20% over this weight range, you are considered by the particular tables to be obese. Sometimes used to determine approximate risk of some cardiovascular diseases, and thus eligibility for certain kinds of insurance.

Ischemia   (is-KEE-me-uh) [From Greek *iskhein,* "to hold back" + *haima,* "blood." From *haima,* we get words like *hemoglobin, hemorrhage,* and *hemorrhoid.*] Decrease in blood supply to your cells due to a constriction or obstruction of the blood vessels, for example during heart attack or muscle spasm. Pain and loss of function follows ischemia.

Ischial Tuberosity   [From Greek *iskhion,* "hip."] Butt bones or sit bones. Protuberance at the base of your lower hip (ischial) bones, where muscles, notably your hamstrings, attach. You can feel your ischial tuberosities as the bumps of bone that you sit on. The ischium is the lowest of the three bones that, together, make up each half of your pelvis. The other bones are the pubic bones, which fuse in front to become your anterior hipbone, and the iliac, whose crests on either side of your hip you can feel as the two "shelves" that you can rest a package upon.

Ischium   [From Greek *iskhion,* "hip joint."] The lowest of the three bones that make up each half of your pelvis. At the bottom of each

ischium is a bump, called the ischial tuberosity, which are the bony
bumps you sit on. *See* Hamstring Muscles, Ilium, Ischial Tuberosity,
and Pubis.

Isotonic [From Greek *isos,* "equal" + *tonos,* "tension."] In chemistry,
a solution containing the same total concentration of dissolved particles as a reference solution, usually your blood or body tissues. For
example, many commercial sport electrolyte drinks are isotonic to
your blood. A popular myth is that your blood is isotonic to sea
water. However, it is much less concentrated, or hypotonic. Even
many sea creatures have different tonicities than the sea. Some are
higher, some lower. They have to constantly pump stuff in or out
to keep their bodies within normal levels.

J

Jiggle Test An informal test of body composition. Jump in the air.
When you land see how long it takes for all your parts to stop
jiggling. Higher times indicate higher fat amounts. *See* Apples and
Pears, Body Mass Index, Calipers, and Hydrostatic Weighing,

K

Krebs Cycle [Named for Sir Hans Adolf Krebs, who won the Nobel
Prize in 1953 for this important discovery.] A cyclic series of reactions
that are part of how you use oxygen to make the energy-yielding
molecule ATP. It is a cycle, as the last step in the chain of reactions
is making the chemical you started with (citric acid). Each of the
steps in the cycle needs a specific enzyme. The electrons removed
during the Krebs cycle enter the second major aerobic pathway to
make ATP energy, called the electron transport chain. The Krebs
cycle is also called the citric acid cycle or tricarboxylic acid cycle
(TCA). *See* Adenosine Triphosphate (ATP), Aerobic Metabolism, and
Electron Transport Chain.

L

Lactic Acid or Lactate [From Latin *lact,* "milk," named because bacteria
in milk produce it from the milk sugar lactose in the process of
making their energy. They excrete the lactic acid into the milk, which
sours it.] Molecule formed by metabolizing glucose for energy, when
there is not enough oxygen present (anaerobic metabolism). Lactic

acid is associated with the burning feeling of muscles that occurs during anaerobic metabolism. When enough oxygen is present, lactic acid changes back to pyruvic acid, which can be used in aerobic metabolism. *See* Anaerobic Capacity, Anaerobic Metabolism, Adenosine Triphosphate (ATP), Glycolysis, and Pyruvic Acid.

Ligament [From Latin *ligare,* "to bind."] Tough, fibrous bands connecting bones to each other, connecting cartilage at a joint, or supporting an organ.

Low-Density Lipoprotein Cholesterol Popularly called "bad cholesterol." Compound containing lipid (fat) and protein. Dietary cholesterol and cholesterol made in your liver are transported to your blood vessels and muscles by LDL. Too much LDL can be a risk factor for cardiovascular disease. *See* Cholesterol and High-Density Lipoprotein Cholesterol.

Lumbar Vertebrae or Lumbar Spine [From Latin *lumbus,* "loin."] The five spinal bones of your lower back. They are named, from top to bottom, L1–L5. The intervertebral discs most often involved in low back pain are between L4 and L5 and, particularly, between L5 and S1. S1 is the first sacral vertebra. *See* Cervical Vertebrae, Disc, Sacrum, and Thoracic Vertebrae.

M

Ma Huang [From Mandarin Chinese *ma,* "hemp" + *huang,* "yellow."] Asian plants of the genus Ephedra, particularly *E. sinica,* which contains the stimulant ephedrine. Ma huang is often sold in health food and oriental medicine stores in various drinks and pills for its stimulant effects on your nervous system, heart, and blood vessels, giving a "peppy" feeling. It can be dangerous in excessive amounts. *See* Ergogenic Aids and Sympathomimetic.

Meniscus [From Greek *meniskos,* diminutive of *mene,* "moon," for its shape.] In anatomy, menisci are flat cartilaginous discs that act as cushions between the ends of your knee bones. In each knee you have two menisci, side-by-side between your upper leg bone (femur) and lower leg bone (tibia). The meniscus on the inner side of each knee is your medial meniscus. The one on the outer side is your lateral meniscus. Menisci can be torn by twisting your knee, and worn out by poor leg postures when walking. *See* Disc.

Metabolism [From Greek *metaballein,* "to change."] The total of all physical and chemical processes in cells and living systems as a whole, necessary for energy synthesis to maintain life.

Menopause [From Greek *meno,* "month" + Greek *pausis,* "cessation."]

The phase of life after menstrual and reproductive functions. Twenty-five percent of all American women reach menopause by age 47, half by 50, three quarters by 52, and 95% by age 55. Menopause is a risk factor for osteoporosis. There seems to be a physical corollary in men, where hormonal functions taper and bone loss accelerates, among other effects.

Minerals [From Latin *mineralis,* pertaining to mines and mining.] Dietary minerals are inorganic elements essential to the health of humans, animals, and plants. Examples are iron, calcium, potassium, sodium, and zinc.

Mole [From German *mol,* short for *Molekulargewicht,* "molecular weight."] A unit of measure to manage large numbers of atoms, molecules, ions, etc. One mole is 6.0225×10^{23}, or Avogadro's number. Also called gram molecule.

Muscle Spindles [Named for their thin, spindle-like shape.] Small, thin, sensory organs in your muscles (and the muscles of all vertebrates). Muscle spindles are very sensitive to the stretch of the muscle they are in. Also called neuromuscular spindle, stretch receptor, and Kühne's spindle. Named for Wilhelm (Willy) F. Kühne, German physiologist and histologist (1837–1900), who first identified them. *See* Myotatic Reflex and Proprioceptors.

Myotatic Reflex [From Greek *myo,* "muscle" + *tasis,* "stretching."] Quick muscle contraction in response to a sudden stretching force on the muscle. Initiated by stimulation of muscle proprioceptors called spindles—stretch receptors in your muscles. Also called the Liddell-Sherrington reflex, the muscular reflex, and the stretch reflex. *See* Muscle Spindles and Proprioceptors.

N

Neurotransmitter [Neuro is from the Greek *sinew,* meaning "string" or "nerve" + transmitter.] A group of chemicals your body produces to send nerve impulses from one nerve ending to the next, across a tiny space called a synapse. Examples of neurotransmitters, among many, are acetylcholine, serotonin, and catecholamines such as dopamine, norepinephrine, and epinephrine.

O

Ondine's Curse (or Undine's Curse) Literary term from Greek mythology for sleep apnea. Ondine (or Undine) was a water sprite who cursed a deserving villain with being only able to breathe voluntarily. When he fell asleep, he stopped breathing, and suffocated. *See* Sleep Apnea.

Oophorectomy (oo-for-EK-tuh-mee) [From Greek *oon,* "egg," + *phoros,* "bearing," + *ectom,* "excising" or "removing."] Surgical removal of the female gonads, the ovaries. Sometimes done in conjunction with a hysterectomy—removal of the uterus. Equivalent in hormonal effect to male castration. A risk factor for osteoporosis.

Osmotic Thirst One of your two thirst mechanisms. Stimulated by high blood electrolyte content, regardless of your body's total water volume. That is why salty things make you thirsty, even when you are drinking (and why bars serve you salty finger food). *See* Hypovolemic Thirst.

Osteomalacia [From Greek *osteon,* "bone" + *malakia,* "softness."] Gradual softening and bending of bone, usually from Vitamin D deficiency. Associated with varying amounts of pain.

Osteopenia [From Greek, *osteon,* "bone" + *penia,* "poverty."] Any decrease in bone mass below normal. Among the causes are osteomalacia and osteoporosis.

Osteoporosis (ah-stee-oh-pore-OH-sis) [From Greek *osteon,* "bone" + *poros,* "passage," "pore" +-*osis,* a condition, from the Greek word for "suffering."] Decreased bone mass leading to porous and fragile bones that fracture easily. At-risk sites are the upper back, hip, and wrist. Healing is difficult and slow. Occurs mainly in postmenopausal women, and elderly men. Important to prevention is resistive exercise, like weight lifting, and resisting your own body weight during weight-bearing exercise like walking, dancing, running, skating, and skiing.

Overload Principle Term to describe the need for greater than accustomed loads to improve exercise capacity. The type of overload required is specific to the system, for example, to increase strength, you need to lift heavier weights (your muscles must contract at tensions close to their maximum). To increase endurance, you need to cover longer distances. To increase your flexibility, you need to regularly take your joints through greater ranges of motion.

Oxygen Debt A term used as if synonymous with oxygen deficit. Refers to the extra oxygen you use during recovery from exercise to "repay" the oxygen needed but not available at the time of high-intensity exercise. When energy stores decrease and lactic acid builds during the "debt" phase, you have to slow or stop exercise, and gasp for more oxygen while your limbs burn with lactic acid. The oxygen you take in during the "debt-paying" phase is used to make energy and remove lactic acid. *See* Anaerobic Capacity and Lactic Acid.

P

Parasympathetic Nervous System   Part of the autonomic nervous system. Works to decrease heart rate, decrease blood pressure, dilate blood vessels, and stimulate digestive secretions. Inhibits or opposes the sympathetic nervous system. The parasympathetic nervous system nerves originate in the brain stem and the lower part of the spinal cord. *See* Sympathetic Nervous System.

Perfusion   [From Latin *perfundere*, "to pour."] Blood flow.

Periosteum   (per-ee-OSS-tee-um) [From Greek *peri*, "around" + *osteon*, "bone."] Membrane that covers your bones except at the bone ends. At bone ends you have cartilage called articular cartilage. The periosteum is an attachment for your muscles and tendons. In young bones, the periosteum has two layers—the inner one makes new bone tissue, and the outer one is the tough, fibrous connective tissue layer that conveys the blood vessels and nerves supplying the bone. As you get older, your inner, bone-producing (osteogenic) layer gets thinner. *See* Bones, Cortical Bone, and Trabecular Bone.

Physiology   [From Greek *phusis*, "nature" + *ology*, "study."] Study of the functions of living beings and their parts.

Pickwickian Syndrome   Informal, literary name for sleep apnea in obese people, named after the "fat boy" in Dickens' *Pickwick Papers*, who was obese with daytime sluggishness. *See* Sleep Apnea.

Plantarflex   [From Latin *plantaris*, from *planta*, "sole of the foot."] To bend the ankle so that the foot points toward the sole, or bottom. *See* Dorsiflex.

Plasma   [From Greek *plassein*, "to mold."] Clear, yellowish, noncellular, fluid part of blood. Makes up about 55% of blood volume. Plasma without the clotting protein fibrinogen is called serum.

Poikilotherm   (POY-kill-oh-thurm) [From Greek *poikilos*, various + *therme*, "heat."] Animals, such as fish and reptiles, whose body temperature varies depending on surrounding temperature. Sometimes called ectotherms. *See* Homeotherms.

Postmenopausal   After menopause. A woman is considered postmenopausal when she has had no menses for one year. *See* Menopause.

Power   [From Latin *potere*, "to be able."] In exercise physiology, power is a measure of how fast you can be strong. Exercise power is the combination of speed and strength. Someone who can lift a weight in 2 seconds has twice the power of someone who needs 4 seconds to move that same weight.

Prime Mover Muscle or muscles mainly responsible for a particular movement.

Premenopausal Before menopause. *See* Menopause.

Proprioceptors [From Latin *proprius,* "one's own or self," + *ceptors,* "receiving information."] Sensory receptors in muscles, tendons, joints, and your inner ear. Proprioceptors detect changes in your position or movement. Your most abundant proprioceptors are your muscle spindles, which notice stretch in your muscles. When suddenly stretched, or stretched too far, your spindles send a signal that stimulates another signal that comes back to tell your muscle to contract. Proprioceptors help you keep your balance, and prevent muscle tears from too much stretch. Also called mechanoreceptors. *See* Myotatic Reflex.

Protein [From Greek *pratos,* "first."] Large, complex, organic molecules of one or more chains of amino acids. Proteins are fundamental components of all living cells, and necessary for proper functioning. Proteins contain carbon, hydrogen, oxygen, nitrogen, and usually sulfur. Many important body components are proteins, such as enzymes, hormones, and antibodies.

Pubis or Pubic Bone [From Latin *pubes,* "groin."] The front, lower part of your hipbones, that form the front arch of your pelvis. The left and right pubic bones come together in front at the pubic symphysis. The pubic bone is distinct at birth and later fuses together with the other two hipbones, the ilium and ischium. *See* Ilium and Ischium.

Pyruvic Acid or Pyruvate [From Greek *pyr(o),* "fire," "heat," or derived from acid + Latin *uva,* "grape" (from being produced by the dry distillation of racemic acid, originally derived from grapes).] Molecule produced from breaking down glucose to make energy (glycolysis). When there is enough oxygen present for the intensity of exercise (aerobic glycolysis), pyruvate can change into another substance called acetyl-CoA, which feeds into your aerobic metabolism where you can make much more energy. When there isn't enough oxygen (during anaerobic glycolysis), pyruvate turns to lactate (or lactic acid). In this case, energy is limited, and the lactate building in your working muscles causes a burning feeling. *See* Aerobic, Glycolysis, and Lactic Acid.

Q

Q$_{10}$ Effect   The enzyme reactions in your cells that produce energy and control body functions speed up as your body temperature rises. A 10° C rise would double the rate of enzyme reactions. This is called the Q10 Effect. Your internal temperature could never change 10° without severe health consequences, but the 2–4 degrees that a warm-up raises your temperature uses the Q$_{10}$ Effect to boost athletic performance, make stretching safer, and soothe arthritic joints.

S

Sacrum   [From Latin *sacrum,* "sacred" (bone).] Broad, slightly curved, triangular bone forming the back wall of your pelvis. Made of five fused vertebrae. It joins the lowest lumbar vertebra from above, the coccyx below, and the hipbones on either side.

Scoliosis   [Greek *skolios,* "crooked"+ the suffix -*osis,* "condition."] Sideways curving or twisting of the spine. There may be one or more curves, and may be due to muscle and/or bone deformity, or due to chronic unequal muscle contractions. Associated pain can often be reduced with good back exercises.

Sleep Apnea   Sleep disorder involving snoring, where the snorer stops breathing during sleep because of upper airway obstruction, causing repeated shortage of oxygen to the brain. Sleep apnea sufferers are often overweight, heavy necked males, but heavy females are also affected. Sleep apnea raises the incidence of stroke and cardiac irregularities. The repeated awakenings from the apnea, sometimes hundreds per night, result in chronic daytime sleepiness. This sleepiness is documented to greatly raise the risk of serious automobile accidents. Sleep apnea can be stopped, but not cured, using high-pressure air that opens airways, delivered by face mask worn during sleep. The machine is called a Continuous Positive Air Pressure (CPAP) machine. For long-term treatment, losing weight is often very effective.

Somatotyping   Body classification system according to three characteristics—thinness or ectomorphy, fatness or endomorphy, and muscularity or mesomorphy. Nobody is only one type, but a combination of them, usually with one or two predominating.

Spondylolisthesis   (spon-di-lo-lis-THEE-sis) [From Greek *spondylo* + *olisthsis,* "slipping and falling."] Slipping, resulting in abnormal forward movement, of one of the vertebrae on the vertebra below it. Sometimes associated with low back pain. Although the bones may not move back into place, the pain is often easily relieved with regular back exercises.

Spot Reducing   Any method thought to remove fat from only specific body areas. Although there are many products and potions on the market promising spot reduction of body fat, only liposuction works.

Sprain   Partial or complete tear of a ligament, from stretching past its limit of range. Usually painful.

Strain   [From Latin *stringere,* "to extend" (and from which we may get the word *perestroika).*] To injure a muscle, sometimes from overuse, sometimes from stretching past its limits.

Strength   [From Old English *strang,* "strong."] Ability to move a heavy weight one or few times.

Stroke Volume (SV).   Amount of blood ejected from the heart with each beat. Stroke volume times heart rate is cardiac output, or SV $\times$ HR = Q. If stroke volume increases with increased venous return, as with immersion or lying down, heart rate decreases to keep cardiac output constant.

Swimmer's Ear   Painful infection or inflammation of the outer ear, which is the part you can see (the auricle) and stick your finger into (the canal). Cotton swabs and scratching the canal contribute to swimmer's ear by removing protective cerumen (ear wax). Ear plugs rarely keep water out, and often create conditions good for swimmer's ear, by rubbing away wax, and holding water in the canal. Swimmer's ear usually is easily prevented and treated with white vinegar or Otic Domeboro drops. Swimmer's ear is not related to middle ear or inner ear injuries caused by pressure, or to congestion of the middle ear, so decongestants do not help. Swimmer's ear does not automatically require stopping swimming or diving, just drying the ears afterward. Serious and recurring cases need medical intervention.

Sympathetic Nervous System   [From Greek *sympatheo,* "to feel with."] Part of your autonomic nervous system. Works to increase heart rate and blood vessel constriction, and reduce digestive secretions. Opposes and balances the parasympathetic nervous system. The sympathetic nervous system nerves originate in the thoracic and lumbar regions of the spinal cord. *See* Parasympathetic Nervous System, and Sympathomimetic.

Sympathomimetic   (sim-path-oh-my-MET-ik) [From *sympatho,* for the sympathetic nervous system + *mimikos,* "imitating."] A substance that mimics the action of your sympathetic nervous system by releasing nerve transmitter chemicals called catecholamines (especially epinephrine and norepinephrine) from nerve endings. Commonly known sympathomimetic substances are amphetamines, ephedrine (found in "health food" stimulants and certain allergy medicines), phenylephrine (powerful vasoconstrictor used in preparations to relieve nasal congestion and maintain blood pressure during anesthesia), and phenylpropanolamine (used as a nasal decongestant, a bronchodilator, and appetite suppressant). The term *adrenomimetic* has been proposed to replace the term *sympathomimetic,* which some feel to be less accurate. Adrenomimetic (add-REE-no-my-MET-ik) means having an action similar to that of the body chemicals epinephrine and norepinephrine. In general, the term *sympathomimetic* is used rather loosely, but should be used only when discussing drugs that actually produce effects that mimic activation of the entire sympathetic system, not just central nervous system stimulation. Not everything that is a central nervous system stimulant is sympathomimetic, for example caffeine, nicotine, strychnine, and picrotoxin. Strychnine and picrotoxin are such strong central nervous system stimulants that they are considered convulsants. *See* Amphetamines, Ergogenic Aid, Ma Huang, and Sympathetic Nervous System.

T

Tendon　[From Latin *tendere,* "to stretch." This derivation is interesting, as tendons don't stretch greatly except with injury.] Tough, fibrous, inelastic modification of the ends of muscle, which connect your muscles to your bones.

Thoracic Vertebrae　[From Latin *thorax,* "breastplate" or "chest."] Twelve upper back bones, named T1 to T12, from upper to lower. A pair of ribs attaches to each thoracic vertebra, 12 pairs of ribs in all. Both men and women have 12 paired ribs, 24 total. Men do not have one less rib.

Trabecular Bone　(tra-BECK-you-lar) [From Latin, diminutive of *trabs,* "beam."] Spongy, branching, supporting meshwork of bone found mostly in your vertebrae and the ends of long bones. Decreased density first occurs in trabecular bone.

U

Undine's Curse　Alternate spelling for Ondine's Curse. *See* Ondine's Curse and Sleep Apnea.

V

Vasoconstriction [From Latin *vas,* "vessel" + Latin *constrict,* "to compress."] Decrease in diameter of blood vessels, usually arterioles.

Vasodilation [From Latin *vas,* "vessel" + Latin *dilatare,* "to enlarge."] Increase in diameter of blood vessels, usually arterioles.

Veins Membranous, branching system of thin-walled tubes that carry blood from all areas of the body back to the heart for transport to the lungs. *See* Arteries.

Vertebra (plural vertebrae) [From Latin *verto,* "to turn."] Spine bone. In humans there are usually 33 vertebrae, 7 cervical (C1–C7), 12 thoracic (T1–T12), 5 lumbar (L1–L5), 5 sacral (fused into one bone, the sacrum), and 4 coccygeal (fused into one bone, the coccyx). Each vertebra bears the weight of all your body above it.

Vitamins [From Latin *vita,*"life" + amine, so called because they were originally thought to be amines.] Any of various organic substances essential for normal growth and activity. Deficiencies may cause various diseases and problems, but taking above a needed amount has not been shown to have beneficial effects. It is often difficult to determine a "needed amount," making the topic difficult to study.

VO$_{2max}$ (pronounced vee-oh-tu-max) VO$_2$ is how much oxygen you consume. The max VO$_2$ is the maximum amount of oxygen your system can extract and use to do exercise.

W

Warm-up Raising your body temperature until it is more energy efficient, and safer for your joints and cardiovascular health to exercise. Best accomplished with a slow, gradual increase in physical activity of the large limbs, as with walking, cycling, and slow jogging. Can also be assisted by passive heating with hot baths and local heat packs.

Waist-to-Hip Ratio A simple, general test of physical status. Take your waist and hip measurements. Divide the waist by the hip measurement. For health, stay below 0.8 for women and 1.0 for men.

Weight-Bearing Activity Exercise where body weight provides the resistance, as in walking, running, dancing, skiing, skating, and hiking. Regular weight-bearing exercise is known to increase bone density and reduce risk of osteoporosis in the hip and back. You need to add weight lifting (or push-ups) to increase bone density at the third site that is most at risk for osteoporosis, the wrist.

Weight-Loading Activity Exercise where external weight provides the resistance, as in weight lifting and carrying packages. Regular weight loading is known to increase bone density and reduce risk of osteoporosis.